PANDORA PRESS HEALTH REPORT

THE PATIENT PATIENTS

Helen Roberts is Senior Researcher at Bradford and Ilkley Community College. Her books include *Miscarriage* (with Ann Oakley and Ann McPherson). She has a young son and lives in Yorkshire.

Helen Roberts

THE PATIENT PATIENTS

Women and Their Doctors

PANDORA PRESS

LONDON · BOSTON · MELBOURNE · AND · HENLEY

First published in 1985
by Pandora Press (Routledge & Kegan Paul plc)

14 Leicester Square, London WC2H 7PH, England

9 Park Street, Boston, Mass. 02108, USA

464 St Kilda Road, Melbourne,
Victoria 3004, Australia and

Broadway House, Newtown Road,
Henley on Thames, Oxon RG9 1EN, England

Set in Sabon
by Columns Ltd, Reading, Berks.
and printed in Great Britain
by Cox and Wyman Ltd,
Reading, Berks.

Library of Congress Cataloging in Publication Data

Roberts, Helen, 1949-

The patient patients.
Bibliography: p.
Includes index.
1. Physician and patient. 2. Women—Medical care.
I. Title.
R727.3.R63 1985 610'.88042 84-22732

British Library CIP data also available

ISBN 0-86358-019-X (p/b)

Contents

Preface and acknowledgments

This book draws much of its illustration from a study of women and their doctors, and therefore owes an enormous debt to those women and doctors who freely gave their time to be interviewed, who agreed to let us look at their medical records, and who allowed us to sit in on consultations. The study was originally a joint one conducted by Michèle Barrett and myself, and I am particularly grateful to her, both for intellectual support in setting up the project and for her part in the fieldwork. In accordance with our assurances of confidentiality, names of patients, doctors and places have been omitted or changed, as have other details which might enable patients or doctors to be individually identified. This means, unfortunately, that those who 'tell' of their experience, rather than write their thoughts, do not get properly acknowledged. I did try using changed names throughout, but this only added to the confusion, since most names one is likely to choose are also the names of real people, who may (wrongly) feel that they have been identified.

Since this is not an academic book, details of the study (and some of the stories involved in setting it up and its progress) appear in an appendix, as do notes, references and more detailed suggestions for reading on some of the topics covered. The main provenance for the ideas in this book is less easy to acknowledge formally by notes and references. This is (in the terms of the American sociologist Pauline Bart) that body of knowledge on the knowledge of bodies which has emerged – or re-emerged – from the women's movement over the last fifteen years or so.

My former secretary, Sue Sinclair, aided the production of this book not by typing the manuscript, but by watching over my work in general while the book was in progress and I was on maternity leave. The final manuscript was expertly prepared by Ellen Taylor, Gerry Rush-Widdup, Shirley Middlemiss and Sue Montague. Monique Crochard, Tracey Turpin and especially Rodney Barker ensured that the progress of this book was not interrupted too often (they claim at all) by domestic labour: Hilary Graham, Ellen Jespersen, Carsten Jespersen, Ian Stanley and Rodney Barker all read the book and made extremely helpful comments, many of which have been incorporated into the text, although probably they would all have liked to see more changes, and shouldn't therefore take any blame for the book's deficiencies. Julia Vellacott was a constructive, helpful and insightful editor, as was Philippa Brewster from Pandora. Carol Gardiner was a patient and considerate copy editor. The ultimate responsibility for the product rests with me.

The birth of my son, Benjamin Barker, delayed the delivery of the manuscript, but brought me into close contact with the medical profession; something which has inevitably affected the course of this book. In particular, it has shown me just how difficult it is to remain in control in the face of the expertise of doctors.

Pandora's advance on the book helped to finance my maternity leave. If you have a manuscript up your sleeve, I suggest you send it to them.

Helen Roberts

Chapter 1

Women, the patient patients

'The consultant was like Jekyll and Hyde in a way. The first year that I was here, I had to go to the hospital every single day for treatment. And, well, I can't say that he was particularly pleasant. But then, when I had this other trouble the doctor said to me, "Well, you need to see the gynaecologist, but there's a ten-month waiting list." Well, this was in February, so the doctor says, "Why not ask the old man?" (he always calls my husband the old man). "Why not ask the old man if you can go private?" So I came home and asked him and straightaway, he rang up the doctor and said yes, he'd pay. Well, that was on the Wednesday, and the gynaecologist saw me on the Friday at his house, and he was *charming*. He was never like that when I saw him at the hospital. It's not right, I suppose, but oh, he was nice.'[1]

'He was that kind, it choked me.'

'If it hadn't been for my GP I wouldn't be here today. He's a marvellous doctor because you can talk and he'll listen.'

'I would say that she is defrosting and just as the fridge always seems to drip a lot when it is defrosting, this lady was dripping a little when I saw her, but then all my ladies drip so I am quite used to that.' (A psychiatrist of his woman patient.)

> 'He's a right vet. . . .' (Middle-aged woman patient of her GP.)

Women go to the doctors more often than men, they take more medicines than men, and they spend more time looking after other people's health than men do. But women and doctors (even if those doctors are women) don't just have subtly different viewpoints about health; they inhabit different worlds.[2] Doctors have the power to define what is, and what is not, illness; what is, and what is not, appropriate behaviour in a patient; and what is to go on in the consulting room.

Doctors and patients alike might be shocked at the suggestion that the doctor–patient relationship is a power relationship. It is only when confronted as a patient with the ability of the doctor to define, to make decisions, to reveal or not to reveal information about health matters which intimately affect ourselves and our children that this power becomes clear. But the power of medicine and the power of doctors over women goes far deeper than the consultation. As Ehrenreich and English point out:[3]

> Medical science has been one of the most powerful sources of sexist ideology in our culture. Justifications for sexual discrimination – in education, in jobs, in public life – must ultimately rest on the one thing that differentiates women from men: their bodies. Theories of male superiority ultimately rest on biology.
>
> Medicine stands between biology and social policy, between the 'mysterious' world of the laboratory and everyday life.

To suggest that such a view is an anachronism is to ignore the reality. In the last century, the exclusion of women from education was justified by a 'concern' for their health. Now, it is being suggested that sexual equality may make women sicker. A recent article in the *Wall Street Journal*,[4] entitled 'Cost of Equality? Women's Problems Grow More Like Men's', discusses an increase in cigarette use, heart disease, car accidents, suicide, a decrease in the rate of women's life expectancy, and an increase in female crime, as well as an increase in female alcoholism:

> In the wake of the revolution in sex roles, and gains in female employment, women are increasingly afflicted by a range of social and physical problems that used to be largely the domain of men. It is a phenomenon that some describe – in a much disputed analysis – as 'the dark side of female emancipation.'

To be fair, in spite of the title of the article and the subtitles ('Gaps between Sexes Narrow in Alcoholism, Suicide, Crime, Even Car Crashes', and 'Stresses of the Working Wife'), space is given to some of the arguments against such an interpretation of the statistics. But the message is clear. Seek equality and you'll get sick. Get a job and drop dead. Equality means problems.

Nothing could demonstrate more clearly how the presentation of health and illness continues to be viewed in terms of interests and assumptions which have nothing whatsoever to do with 'purely medical' criteria, if such criteria could be imagined. A problem for men – that women are after 'men's jobs' and are increasingly reluctant to support men's careers by unpaid labour in the household – is presented as a problem for women. From the Tower of Babel onwards, confusion and pestilence have been threatened as the awful consequence of the aspirations of the oppressed. And women, of course, are not the only oppressed group, nor the only group whose status and aspirations are dealt with through the language and constraints of medicine. Wider and wider aspects of all our lives are becoming medicalised. Irving Zola[5] talks about the way in which the labels 'healthy' and 'ill' are now seen as being relevant to a greater and greater part of human existence. Others, looking at the use of drugs have pointed to the 'renaming and relabelling as medical problems calling for drug intervention a wide range of human behaviours which, in the past, have been viewed as falling within the bounds of the normal trials and tribulations of human existence.'[6] In a society where every day more than half the adult population and nearly one-third of the children take or use some kind of medicine,[7] the power of doctors and pharmaceutical companies is enormous.

At the level of the individual consultation, it can be difficult to recognise what is going on – especially if we have a doctor we like, who is hard working, pleasant and kind. But putting it at its most simple level, how often, particularly in hospital, have *you* been called by your first name by the medical staff? Perhaps the doctors are just being friendly, but they aren't usually so friendly that you can call the doctor Fred. However good an individual doctor is and however assertive an individual patient, one of them is in charge, and it's not the patient.

Of course, it may sometimes seem to the doctor as she is interrupted for the third time when reading her children's bedtime story, or he's called out of his bed for the fourth time in a week, that the power is the other way round, or that power is simply another word for responsibility. But is it? This book argues that women patients could get a better deal and that all of us, doctors and patients alike, would benefit from change. The quotations from women and doctors at the start of this chapter show some of the problems. Women *want* to like their doctors, and they want to give them the benefit of the doubt if things aren't quite right. The patient at the beginning of the chapter, for instance, was appreciative of the consultant's courtesy when he was paid a direct fee rather more than she was critical of his lack of it when she saw him as an NHS patient.

Many, probably most, doctors do the best possible job for their patients within the terms set for the relationship. But how good is that relationship? This isn't an anti-doctor book, but that doesn't mean that doctors will see it as 'fair'. The doctor–patient relationship isn't a 'fair' one. What this book does is to illustrate some of the hidden dimensions of power between doctors and their women patients and to suggest what might be done to redress the balance.

Doctors are important to women both symbolically and in real life. Many public libraries have a 'Doctor and Nurse' romance section; TV series about doctors are sure-fire winners. We don't have long television series on *Garage Mechanic Kildare*, or *Tax Inspector's Casebook*. By why are doctors so special? Why is it necessary to write about the relationship of women with their doctors? And is this relationship any more important than the relationship we might have with other people in our everyday lives – our children's teachers, the health visitor, the dentist?

One of the reasons why the relationship is so important for

women is the fact that women are dependent on medicine and doctors for the most basic control of their own bodies. It often seems that the power of reproduction – of getting or not getting pregnant, staying or not staying pregnant, having a baby – is as much in the doctor's province as in the mother's.

But although every woman has a story about her doctor, little has been written on the intimate world of relationships and feelings about doctors from the patient's point of view. Patients tend to be presented as problems for doctors, rather than the reverse. While the subject of doctor–patient communication is of growing interest to some of those within the medical profession, most of the literature in this area is written for the doctor and from his or her viewpoint. In one crucial area, that of childbirth, and thanks largely to the works of feminists, we do know something about the feelings of 'patients' and, what is more, this work has had wide-ranging effects. If enough customers are unhappy, if enough beds are empty in particular maternity hospitals, if enough women complain, then even the most intransigent of physicians feel compelled at least to think about the service they are providing. (Whether they publicly acknowledge the reasons for their reappraisal is another matter.)

A sociologist doing work on GPs found that women patients frequently fell into the category of 'most trouble'.[8] At the same time, although health is difficult to measure, women tend to consider themselves more unhealthy than do men, and women go to the doctor more often than men.[9] In the 15–44 age group, women go twice as often, though this is of course the age group where women are particularly likely to attend for contraceptive or ante-natal care. But even in other age groups, women are more prone to go to the doctor.

As Princess Anne so charmingly put it, becoming a mother is one of the occupational hazards of being a wife, and becoming a mother, or avoiding becoming one, sets off a whole train of visits to the doctor's surgery. Women go to the doctor not only on their own behalf, but, to a greater extent than men, they go for their spouse, their children, their aged parents, or even for their neighbours. Women, when questioned, admit to feeling unhealthy more often than men do, and yet they live longer. What might explain this? Constance Nathanson[10] has given three main explanations for sex differences in illness. First, it may be that women admit to or report more illness than men for the reason that it's more acceptable in our culture for women to say that they're ill, particularly with minor illnesses. Second, being ill (or adopting what sociologists call the 'sick role') may be more compatible with a woman's other responsibilities than with a man's responsibilities. A working man has to make a decision about whether or not to go on working, with considerable financial implications. So long as a woman's work is in the home or largely in the home, she can struggle on. Finally, of course, it may well be that women report more ill-health and go to the doctor more often because they are sicker than men. Although we commonly think that men die earlier than women because they have more stressful lives, it could just as easily be the case that it is the more stressful lives that women lead which send them to the doctor so often.

Two American sociologists[11] have suggested some explanations for the fact that women, especially married women, more often become mentally ill then men. (Mental 'illness' is itself not without problems of definition, which we will return to later.) They suggest that married women's roles are particularly frustrating, and give five possible reasons for women's emotional problems. First, housewives tend to have no alternative sources of gratification outside the family (and as Chapter 5 which deals with the family indicates, this may also be true of women who work outside the home). Second, housework is seen as being unskilled and having little prestige ('I'm only a housewife'). Third, the lack of structure in the housewife's day may give her time to brood over troubles. Fourth, working wives have, on the whole, less satisfactory jobs than men, and going out to work places them under more strain than men, since they also have work to do in the home. Finally, the sorts of expectations we have of women as women, wives, mothers or workers are generally ambiguous and conflicting. These explanations are not altogether satisfactory, and are better in any case at explaining women's greater tendency to illness than they are at explaining their tendency to live longer, but they provide a starting-point for understanding the problem.

But women are not just 'consumers' of health care. They are

also 'producers' of good health – the good health of their children, their husbands, their elderly parents.[12] Women as mothers, as wives, as daughters, as friends, as neighbours, tend to be the first port of call for people who are feeling ill. Many illnesses never get to the doctor at all, but are dealt with in the home. The fact that most of these illnesses are minor ones doesn't make the job of looking after the sick person any less of a job. Women may not be taking out the appendix, treating the duodenal ulcer, stripping the varicose veins, but they are doing the bulk of health care in our society, the bulk of preventative work and, possibly, even giving the bulk of advice. This advice is so much a part of our everyday lives that we hardly even see it as advice: 'Don't eat that, Sam, it will rot your teeth,' 'Try rubbing in some oil to get rid of his cradle cap,' 'A dry biscuit in the morning first thing when I was pregnant used to stop me feeling so sick. Why not try that?' There is, though, a real cold war over women as producers of knowledge about health care. Doctors have long warned us about going to another woman for advice. 'Old wives' tales' are dangerous. As one booklet written for women advises:[13]

> She should be chary of talking overmuch to her friends. . . . They are all too often eager to pass on to her innumerable superstitions on the subject which are never any help and often are a cause of worry. But simple medical treatment . . . may do a world of good. . . . It is silly to struggle on without help when your doctor can help you.

The fact that talking to women friends is seen as struggling on 'without help' reveals a curious contradiction in the attitudes of the medical profession. On the one hand, women are in doctors' 'most trouble' category, because they are seen as making excessive demands. They are consequently advised to deal with minor problems themselves, and there is a deeply embedded notion in most women (whether or not they do go to the doctor a lot) that they shouldn't 'bother' the doctor. On the other hand, doctors are keen to retain their place as experts, knowing more about women and women's bodies than the women do themselves, as the following dialogues from one of Ann Oakley's books[14] illustrate:

DOCTOR (reading case notes): Ah, I see you've got a boy and a girl.

PATIENT: No. Two girls.

DOCTOR: Really, are you sure? I thought it said . . . (checks in case notes) Oh no, you're quite right, two girls.

And again:[15]

MALE DOCTOR: Will you keep a note in your diary of when you first feel the baby move?

PATIENT: Do you know – well, of course, you would know – what it feels like?

MALE DOCTOR: It feels like wind pains – something moving in your tummy.

All this forms a backdrop to a situation where what the patient actually *says* is dismissed as being too subjective to be taken into account. Of course, it is subjective, and she is the subject. As one GP has written (admittedly of her hospital training). '[You get] more prizes for coming up with an interesting quotation from a journal than for knowing how someone is feeling about being ill.'[16] And a feminist writer looking at one of the major studies in Britain on the safety of oral contraceptives pointed out that women's own evidence on headaches, lack of libido, and so on, was considered 'too subjective' to be assessed.[17]

While it is comforting to know that our medical advisers set so much store by 'scientific' evidence (and what a doctor 'knows' seems to be more likely to be considered 'fact' than what a patient 'knows', or what she feels), it is also the case that what a doctor 'knows' has a tendency to change over time. At one time, the medical profession was advising that if women were to study, and especially if they were to study to become doctors, their health (and particularly their reproductive health) would suffer.[18] Until recently, doctors 'knew' that it was a good idea for a woman to give birth lying on her back. Some twenty or so years ago, many doctors 'knew' that children with sore throats should have their tonsils out.

This book is based on the view that what women say about themselves, their doctors, their illnesses and the illnesses of their families is worth listening to. It is particularly important at a time when doctors are not only claiming or being granted expertise over greater and greater areas of everyday life, but also when more and more specialists are claiming expertise over women's bodies.

We can see something of the breadth of expertise claimed by doctors in the Family Doctor booklets, published by the British Medical Association and available quite cheaply from corner chemists. As well as booklets on heart attacks, epilepsy and rheumatism (all part of the doctor's sphere of expertise), there is also a booklet on *Women: The Middle Years* (though not, apparently, a similar one for men), *Marriage: Making or Breaking* and *Teenage Living and Loving*. We can see something of the number of experts claiming expertise on the woman's body from a passage from a recent book about the menopause: 'The peri menopause is emerging more and more as a subject of study by the doctor, the psychologist, the social worker, the gerontologist, the clinical chemist, the public health specialist, the sociologist, the psychiatrist and the experimental pathologist.'[19] The authors are right, of course. It is quite a little cottage industry.

But where are the women in all this, apart from being patient patients? Of course, some of them may *be* doctors, chemists, psychologists or gerontologists, but it's far more likely that they will not be these people, but their patients. It is because patients have an expertise of their own – both as patients and as carers – that much of this book draws so frequently on what they say.

Chapter 2

What do women think of their doctors?

For many, perhaps most, women, their relationship with their doctor is not a trivial matter, and may be emotionally highly charged. 'He's OK,' is a rare response to a request for information about a woman's doctor. The relationship is more likely to be a love–hate one, ranging from adulation to vitriol, as the two examples below indicate.

Mrs D. was a divorced woman living alone and holding down a responsible and well-paid job. She had had a series of health problems, and had spent quite a bit of time at the doctor's. As we sipped sherry in her front room, she described her doctor in unusual terms: 'He's a right vet.' The cause of her dissatisfaction was then unfolded. She had seen a television programme about cervical cancer and had gone to her doctor asking for a smear, which he had refused on the grounds that it was less than three years since her last one. She told the story of this and many other consultations with some relish, and ended maliciously: 'I just hope he takes cancer of the wee John Willy.'

Mrs M. had five children, all now teenagers, she had a cleaning job mornings and evenings, and was a school dinner lady in between. She hardly ever went to the doctor (she probably didn't have time to), but this didn't stop her having an opinion about him:

> 'He's the best, old Dr L., because if you call him, he's there. And you can go down and see him. I know so many people that feel really ill and they've got to make an appointment. And what's more silly than having to make an appointment

and they might not see you for two or three days? To me, that's a bit silly. I know they've got to do that because some people live down there, don't they? I think they go down there just to read the magazines. . . . I've only had Dr L. and before him Dr M. and you couldn't wish for nicer doctors. I mean, old Dr L.'s got the patience of a saint. He sits down and listens to my old mum, and he never gets irritated. He just sits there and smiles and chats away to her. He's very nice to the older people, see. How he finds time, I dunno, 'cause he's always busy.'

Neither Mrs D.'s criticisms, nor Mrs M.'s praise of the GP would have been made to him direct. Experiences with the doctor become woven into 'stories', and as researchers[1] who have written about going to see the doctor have pointed out, stories may be one way in which some redress is made for the inequalities in the relations between doctor and patient. Women normally have more opportunities than men to develop a relationship with their doctor, and this relationship is by no means in the same league as the relationship with the health visitor, the dentist, or even the hairdresser.

What do women think of their doctors? Certainly, the overwhelming majority rarely voice open protest, perhaps partly because to admit to not having a good doctor might be seen as not having made a good choice oneself, or not 'being bothered' to find another. Possibly it is difficult to see how things might be different, since we are so used to an authority relationship with doctors. When patients do talk of bad doctors, what are the themes?

'Bad' doctors

On the whole, 'bad' doctors are never quite 'bad' really. They can always be excused. They are 'clever', 'good with children', 'kind to the old people', 'too busy to be nice'. It was significant that a lot of stories about 'bad' doctors weren't presented as such and, in fact, would be prefaced with remarks such as: 'He's a good doctor, I've nothing against him, but. . . .' The story that followed would indicate that, indeed, as a doctor, there might be little to complain about; it was as a person that there were complaints to be made. Offhandedness, rudeness, not having enough time, writing a prescription as you came in the door – these are all part of being a 'bad' doctor. It was also the locums and the hospital doctors who were most likely to be 'bad'.

Jane S., her husband and her two children live in a neat council house. She is a lively woman who used to enjoy dancing, but is painfully nervous and shy. She has been agoraphobic for the last ten years, and rarely goes beyond the garden gate. She said that she had been afraid of being interviewed, but had agreed because she thought maybe her doctor, Dr T., was in trouble and she could help. She told a story about the partnership between Dr T. and Dr K. One evening when Dr K. had been on duty, her husband had taken her to the surgery to discuss her agoraphobia. Dr K. had said: 'If you don't pull yourself together in two weeks, I'll put you in the mental hospital.' She explained that the partnership, which had been dissolved by the time I spoke with her, had thrown up a lot of problems:

> 'It was ever so embarrassing because, in the end, there'd be a whole lot of people in the waiting room and they'd all be waiting to see Dr T. ['good' doctor] and Dr K. ['bad' doctor] would be sitting there with nothing to do. If they both pushed their bells at the same time, the person would always go to Dr T. Well, once, it was awful, Dr K. – I felt sorry for him – he came out and said, "Doesn't anyone want to see me?" And I'm such a coward that I said that I did. But I didn't really, because he'd said that to me about the mental hospital.'

It was only very occasionally that a doctor would be seen as bad not because of the way he or she behaved with a patient, but because of the way in which a diagnosis was made or a treatment given. Problems raised tended to be: the hand poised over the prescription pad from minute one of the consultation; the refusal to listen to certain symptoms because they were apparently irrelevant to the history from the doctor's point of view; being too willing, or too unwilling, to prescribe. (Some of these will be discussed further in Chapter 3.) But what of the doctor who was much more evident in patients' accounts – the 'good' doctor?

'Good' doctors

Just as it was rare among the patients we spoke to for the 'bad' doctor to be so judged because of dissatisfaction with medical performance, similarly, the criteria for judging the 'good' doctor were not his clinical skills or academic acumen. Studies have been done on what characteristics make up a 'good' patient. We know less about what makes a 'good' doctor from the patient's point of view. And a 'good' doctor from the point of view of the patient may very well be a quite different creature from, for instance, the Royal College of General Practitioners' idea of what makes a good doctor, or the practising doctor's view of what makes a good doctor.

Perhaps the most important difference would be the lack of emphasis patients put on skill – or rather, the emphasis put on social as opposed to medical skills. Presumably, this is not only because patients are not in a position to judge the latter skills, but because, for most consultations, it is the former which are the more important. If a large number of consultations with the GP are related to anxiety and depression, or relatively minor, if troublesome, complaints and the sort of chronic complaint which is contained rather than cured, then what really matters is that the visit to the doctor's should provide reassurance, should be as unthreatening as possible, should be recognised by the GP as being the social as well as the medical encounter which it is. This is not to say, of course, that 'medical' skills aren't important to the GP. Since for most patients he or she is the point of access to any sort of treatment, then missing an acute appendicitis, a rare tropical disease or an early manifestation of cancer could be fatal. It is simply that for most patients, for most of the time, it is not these skills which are required. It would appear that for most patients, a 'good' doctor is a nice doctor – a sensible enough judgment, since few patients are in a position to say, 'His clinical judgment is first rate,' or 'Look at those clever articles he's written in the *BMJ*.' It is striking to see the way in which many patients cunningly manage to slip in references to the niceness or otherwise of their doctor to the most unpromising of questions (such as, 'How has your health been over the past year?').

'Oh, he is a good doctor. Medically speaking, I don't know. But to talk to, you feel as if there's no one been in before you and there's no one following you. It feels as though his time is your time, which is a good thing.' As this woman so rightly points out, it is a doctor's social and not his medical skills which patients are in a position to judge. A recurring theme was the 'good' doctor who had time to listen to you, and a great deal more emphasis was put on his ability to listen than his ability to advise. As one patient said: 'If it hadn't been for the doctor, I wouldn't be here today. He's a marvellous doctor. You can talk and he'll listen.' Another agreed: 'I don't mind if it's a man or a woman doctor, so long as you can get someone who will listen to you.' Again, Mrs A.'s doctor was 'one of the nicest GPs I've ever had, and he's always the same. I don't know what I'd do if I moved. He's really absolute tops.' Another patient pointed out the advantages of a single-handed practice once one had found a good doctor: 'It's rather nice to go to one doctor. . . . He gets to know you better. He's always jolly, never miserable. . . . You might go in and out and wonder why you went in . . . which I'm afraid it is a bit that way these days. But people make it like that. . . . It's packed.'

Perhaps the stereotype of the doctor as a reassuring father figure, but one who might get angry, was brought out by one woman's remark about her GP: 'He doesn't blow his top. He's very tolerant, very tolerant.' The theme of listening, and of the doctor having time for you was taken up by a patient who wrote of her group practice:

> You can go to them for all sorts of aches and pains, and they listen with intent before examining you and if necessary, prescribing drugs for you. You can call our doctors out after surgery hours for children's ailments and emergencies and they always have a smiling face and cheery word. If it's personal problems, then the doctors are still

there to listen and advise, considering them to be as important as medical ones.

It is worth saying that there is some evidence that doctors identified as 'good' by patients do have 'real' medical as well as social payoffs from the treatment they offer. A patient responding to a newspaper article about women and doctors was a case in point:

> I feel I must write and pay a tribute to my doctor who really cares. I was forced to change to him, having moved to another district. My previous doctor, like many others, could only write me a prescription and never took the time to talk to me to try and find out if there was another way we could treat my awful depression. I have been suffering from endometriosis for some years, and my last operation left me helpless and hopeless. I wondered just how long I could carry on life in this way, and my doctor at that time could only prescribe more pills. . . . I felt sick with despair, and the only consolation I had was that there were a lot of other women in the same state. Suddenly my whole life changed with my current doctor. When I consulted him for another routine prescription, he took the time to talk to me. He spent the next hour of his valuable time with me. Although I felt very guilty for taking so much of his time, he assured me that it was part of his job to help me, however long it took to do it, and he wasn't just there to cure physical ailments. He didn't write a prescription as he considered it wasn't necessary, but he did give me one for a new way of life by putting back the confidence I had lost in myself.

In sum, then, top of the list of qualities of a 'good' doctor was a willingness to listen; top of the list of complaints would be a visit where, 'You're in and out, and sometimes you wonder why you've come.' Women spend a good deal of time listening to other people – their husband's day, their children's day. Many, perhaps most, have at least occasionally the experience of being not only invisible, but also inaudible as far as other people are concerned. Being a 'good wife' and a 'good mother' has to do with putting other people's interests first. As an article written as late as 1961 in *Woman's Own* put it:[2]

> Ask any man if he'd rather his wife worked or stayed at home and see what he says. If she is listening, he may echo all her excuses about her job making her a more interesting person. . . . But if you could get him alone, I believe he would tell you he would rather she stayed at home and looked after his children, and was waiting for him with a decent meal and a sympathetic ear when he got home from work . . . men don't want to talk about a woman's work. They want to talk about their own.

No wonder that someone whose job it is to listen is valued. Women who provide a twenty-four-hour-a-day listening, counselling, cleaning, cooking and healing service for others are likely sometimes to need similar services themselves. And even if women don't actually *need* a listener, a woman is the major source of information about her own body and life. A doctor can only tap this source of information by listening.

Men doctors and women doctors

Up to now in this chapter, the doctor has been 'he', the patient 'she'. This is not because there are no women GPs – indeed, one in seven are,[3] including some of the doctors quoted in this book. Most women patients have been treated by a women doctor at some time in their lives, and given that niceness, approachability and having time for you are characteristics valued by patients in a 'good' doctor it would seem likely that women doctors – who, as women, are more likely to have acquired precisely these characteristics – would be the patients' first choice. However, when asked whether they would prefer a man or a woman doctor, most patients claim that the sex of the doctor doesn't matter – in much the same way as some doctors claim that the sex of their patients doesn't matter. Just as some of the doctors we spoke to would say, 'A patient's a patient,' when asked about men and women patients, a good many of the women patients would say, 'A doctor's a doctor.' This, however, sometimes leads on to the remark that they did really prefer a man. Mrs B. said:

> 'I'd always sooner have a man doctor, and now you're going to ask me why. Well, in most cases, I think they're more sympathetic, and I find it easier to talk to a man than to a woman . . . most women are tougher with women. Do you know what I mean by that? I suppose there's the feeling, from my generation anyway . . . the question of efficiency. It's awfully wrong, but it's something that you feel. There were very few women doctors when I was young, you see.'

The question of finding it easier to talk to men was brought up by other patients: 'A woman doctor, I know you can talk to a woman doctor 'cause I've had one, but I don't think you can talk to them as much as a man. I don't know why, I really don't know.'

Some women did say that they preferred a woman for a gynaecological examination. One woman had been embarrassed not so much by being examined by a man as by his calling in a chaperone. She explained:

> 'Well, there again, you see, when I went in about this last trouble, he had to call a woman in. Oh, I got that embarrassed waiting for her to come. No, I prefer a lady I think for this. I've got nothing aginst Dr B. – don't think that. It was just this waiting for this nur . . . no, receptionist to come in. It was a bit awkward, I felt, but he probably wasn't awkward about it. I don't suppose it worried him.'

Other women may experience the same – or an even worse – embarrassment at being examined by a woman. As one patient put it: 'I prefer a man. I can talk to a man. I can speak easier to men. I suppose I feel embarrassed with women. I don't know.' . . .

Not all women feel this way, of course. Among certain ethnic groups, a woman will be the doctor of choice, and the same will probably go for women who have come into contact with the women's movement and feel positively about being treated by a woman doctor. Even in a more general population, one study found that most patients expressed no preference about the sex of the doctor, but where there was a preference, 20 per cent of women preferred a female doctor, and 25 per cent of men a male one; 3 per cent of women expressed a preference for a male doctor.[4] As Ann McPherson, a GP who has written on women's problems in general practice, points outs, men can easily have their wishes met in this respect, but a woman's preference for a woman doctor cannot always be met while only 14 per cent of GPs are women.[5]

It should also be stressed (and this will be discussed further in Chapter 6) that where women provide health care for other women as a positive option – through Well Women Clinics, for instance – women doctors are greatly in demand. This seems to lend weight to the view the the 'package' of health care we are offered needs to be looked at in terms of the context in which it is made available. The same facilities and services may appear quite different to patients – may indeed function quite differently, even in medical terms – depending on whether they are shared, provided, or bestowed. If the context is one of medical expertise and medical power, then however 'good' the doctor might be (and this goes for women as well as men), he or she still holds all or most of the cards, and the patient virtually none. The power relationship between individual patients and doctors can't even begin to be evened out until alterations are made to the general framework of experts who bestow, and patients who receive, medical wisdom and treatment. Possibly, the nature of the medical consultation as a social encounter, the fact that for many women it is a moment when they can put down their guard and be on the receiving rather than the giving end, may go some way towards explaining the reluctance among those middle-aged women we spoke to to go to a woman doctor. It is culturally more acceptable to appear 'weak' in front of a man, and perhaps when visiting a woman doctor, there is always the feeling that she also has children to look after, a husband, a home, problems of her own. What is more, that recognition is coupled with the fact that she is there in the surgery doing a job – emphasising, perhaps, the fact that some women can cope.

Several women felt that women doctors were 'tougher' or 'less sympathetic', and perhaps it is the case that some women doctors come to work to practise medicine and not to utilise those listening, caring and reassuring skills which they are already expending to the full in the home. Gail Young has pointed out in an article describing her own training as a doctor: 'a woman doctor, whatever her job, is seen in our culture as an honorary man, simply by virtue of society's concept of what a doctor is, and she will therefore have a lot of difficulty in integrating her self concept as a woman with her doctoring.'[6] Becoming emotionally involved with patients is actively discouraged in training. Knowing how a patient feels is not the most valued of skills. Nurses care and doctors cure.

A little over a century ago, the editor of the *Lancet* wrote: 'woman as a nurse is the natural help of man as a doctor. Woman as a doctor is a conceit contradictory to nature, and doomed to end in disappointment to both the physician and the sick.'[7] At about the same time, the *British Medical Journal* argued: 'it is scarcely possible for a woman to go through a course of medical education without losing that simplicity and purity of character which we so much value . . . in the truest interest of women, it is better that they should not practise the medical profession.'[8] This did not mean, however, that women's caring skills could be dispensed with: 'We have frequent reason to lament that there is no spinster aunt or sister at hand to take charge of some poor invalid. I cannot think therefore that lack of useful employment can drive many to seek occupation in a sphere outside their own family.'[9]

Are such attitudes out of date? It seems not. A recent article in the *Journal of the Royal College of General Practitioners* on doctors' attitudes to women in medicine found that 'There is only moderate enthusiasm in the medical profession for an increase in the number of women doctors.'[10] Similarly, a recent book on *The Family Doctor*,[11] written by an eminent retired GP, is highly ambivalent on the question of women GPs. While recognising the value of women doctors, the author writes:[12]

> I always worry . . . about families where the wife and mother is a doctor. There is a great need for women doctors in the community and women are so full of gentleness and compassion that they are born for general

> practice. Yet I cannot see how a woman can lead such a life and at the same time be a wife to her husband, and more important, a mother to her children.

The Family Doctor was first published in 1981, by which time over one in seven GPs was a woman, and over one in three trainees in general practice was female.

Given this rather ambivalent attitude towards women doctors by the medical profession at large, it is possible that when women patients complain that women GPs are 'tougher', this could well be because they *are* tougher; they need to be tougher – one of the ways of succeeding as a woman doctor without facing too many conflicts could be by being 'one of the boys', or perhaps by being more one of the boys than the boys themselves. This may well make it more difficult for a woman patient to reconcile herself to being treated by a woman GP.

Another powerful factor may be our own mental image of 'The Doctor'. The common stereotype of a kindly, middle-aged, white man, perhaps greying at the temples and wearing a suit, may be challenged in all sorts of ways – by young doctors, overseas doctors and doctors wearing casual clothes. Perhaps, though, it's the female doctor who challenges it most profoundly, as is evidenced by the following riddle:

> A man is driving along with his son when they are involved in a terrible accident. The father is killed outright, the son seriously injured and taken to hospital. As he is wheeled into the operating theatre, the surgeon looks at the child and says, 'I can't operate. That's my son.' What is the relationship of the surgeon to the boy?

The doctor's a busy man

Many of the factors which influence a woman's pattern of visits to a doctor are material matters: working hours, availability and cost of transport, cost of prescriptions and general inconvenience. One person quoted in the Consumers' Association survey of GPs put it like this: 'You have to know at least four days in advance that you or your child is going to be ill.'[13] But other factors also come into play, particularly 'being fair', fear (of the doctor rather than the illness) and, linked with both these, the idea that 'the doctor's a busy man.' These were the feelings expressed both by patients who often go to the doctor's and by those who go only rarely.

Part of 'being fair' to the doctor is based on anxiety, nervousness, even fear, about going to his surgery. This fear is not, as one might expect, simply a fear of being ill, or seriously ill. It is very often directly related to the receptionist, the waiting, and the doctor himself. One woman who rarely went to the doctor's said:

> I don't sit in the doctor's surgery. I get too scared, I think, wondering if he thought I was bad enough. I think that's the trouble with a lot of women, you know. A lot I've spoke to, my friends. 'Cause I sit there and I rehearse what I'm going to say.

Another admitted: 'I send my husband, he goes for me. I get so scared and het up. I sit in that waiting room and rehearse what I have to say. Well, he is a busy man . . . he's a marvellous bloke.'

The fear that you're going to the doctor's too often, or going with problems which are trivial, is a widespread one: 'I've had all sorts with me back and me ears troubling me. Mind you, I daren't go and see him. If I go on, he'll need a suitcase for me cards.' One woman, who lived next door to the doctor's surgery and was an unusually high attender, put it like this:

> 'If I feel rough, I think, "Oh, I'll call in on the doctor." I don't believe in playing around. If I have something which after a day or two I think I ought to see him, I just go. I think it's no good messing about. You get cured much quicker, don't you?'

In some cases, it would be 'only fair' to treat yourself for as long as possible because 'the doctor's a busy man'; in other cases (the high consulters), it was preferable to get into the doctor's as quickly as possible before the disease had a chance to get a grip. That way, he's got a better chance of effecting a cure. 'Doctoring yourself' was frequently part of being fair, and this would often involve proprietary medicines:

> 'I mean, as I say, if I felt meself a bit off weather, I'd get meself a tonic. Because sometimes, I think, they're good for you. But I wouldn't take them regularly all the time. But I think, sometimes, I think if we're going to have a hard winter, I'll take those halibut oil tablets. If I feel a bit upty-whatsit, I'd go down the chemist and get meself a tonic of some sort, see. Because you can get nice ones. I had one once. Old Dr L. gave it to me once – oh, a couple of years ago when I had that cold, oh, a bad cold I couldn't shake off. And it had seven essential vitamins or something. . . . Now last year, I thought, "Hello, you need a bottle of that," so I went down, got a bottle, and that's it. No more. I might go another year or two years, but if I felt under the weather, that's what I'd do if I thought I needed anything like that.'

This particular patient was a very low attender ('I've been lucky,' she said) and had a preventive health care programme of her own:

> 'If I felt really ill, I'd go down. I'd always go to Dr L. if there was something I was worried about . . . I'd go for these cancer tests, too, because I think that's good for you. I'm not frightened of anything like that. And I goes and gives me pint of blood. So there again, if there was anything wrong with you, they'd soon let you know. It's for me own good, innit?'

Other patients, too, would remember what the doctor had prescribed for them one year, and another time try to get the same thing directly from the chemist so as not to bother the doctor. Mrs T. explained:

> 'I had cystitis last year, and that pulled me down a lot. Then, three weeks ago, I had another attack so I sent my husband along to Parrish and Greens, the chemist, for the same stuff as the doctor gave me last year. I didn't want to bother him.'

Several women, in order to be 'less bother', would save up their complaints; when they felt they had enough to go to the doctor's with, they would make a visit. They would then feel that they were bothering him with too many complaints. One woman said: 'I have to wait until I've got half a dozen complaints before I go and see the doctor.' Another admitted: 'If I know what I feel ill from, I dose meself. Unless I've got to go to the doctor's to renew me nerve tablets, I save up me complaints, and then they usually get better.' Mrs F. was the same: 'I'm inclined to keep putting it off. I think maybe it will go the next day. I don't like to make a fuss, somehow. I suppose it's wrong, but I'm not the type to rush to the doctor's, sort of thing.' Some patients would 'bother' the doctor only under certain circumstances. One said:

> 'Normally, I'd look after meself and if I didn't feel any better in about a week, I'd go down to the doctor's. I do go for my chest, though. I smoke too much, and anything you can buy for it doesn't do as much as what the doctor can give you.'

The woman who spoke to us about their health were middle aged, usually from the suburbs and predominantly described themselves as 'housewives'. This did not mean, however, that they did no work outside the home. Several had two or even three part-time jobs, most had some work outside the home, some fostered children or were childminders. Despite the stereotype of the bored, middle-aged woman patient with time on her hands and nothing better to do than kick her heels for a few hours in a doctor's waiting room, it is clear that, for most women, time is at a premium – plans have to be made for various things to be 'fitted in', and enforced inactivity (waiting to see the doctor, for instance) is difficult to cope with. As one woman put it: 'When you've got five kiddies, you're sort of on the trot all the time . . . but I've always enjoyed it. All I need's a bit more time, and, as I say, a bit more money to buy things.'

There is the occasional complaint about the appointments system that doesn't work, the lack of an appointments system that means you have to wait, and the patients who spend 'hours' with the doctor. Nevertheless, there is a much greater tendency to talk about the fact that the doctor is busy than that you are busy yourself. This is linked to views about when and whether to go to the doctor's. One woman said:

> 'I wouldn't rush to the doctor's. I never have. I . . . I've got this thing, you know. The doctors, they have such a terribly busy life. If I was *really* worried, I have been to the doctor's when I've been really worried about something. But no, I'm not a rusher to the doctor's.'

Another, rarely at the doctor's said: 'I mean, I think the doctor's a busy person, and, I mean, years ago when you had to pay for the doctor, you got over your ailments unless it was something really serious.'

All this adds up to a situation where women, although recognising just how pushed they are themselves for time, are more apt to recognise how busy the doctor is than fully to acknowledge just how busy they are themselves, and what sort of effect this might be having on their health. Caring too much about what your doctor thinks about you may damage your health.

Women and doctors: a power relationship

The power and control aspects of going to see the doctor are rarely recognised as such by either party. Doctor and patient normally agree that the doctor defines the situation, and defines what is and what is not acceptable as appropriate for the patient to talk about. Devices such as interrupting, beginning to write a prescription or starting to conduct the examination, may be used to indicate that what the patient is saying is not important or relevant. It is normally the doctor, too, who defines when the consultation has ended and both sides would be shocked if the consultation were to proceed in any other way. We learn that we should not 'bother' the doctor with trivial problems, that the doctor is a 'busy man', that he can call you Jane but you can't call him Fred. These rules may be operated in different ways by different patients; they are nevertheless rules implicitly, if not explicitly, understood.

The closest the women we spoke to got to talking about a recognition of this power relationship was in their expression of fear about going to the doctor's, and in their concern with being 'fair' to him. As one woman pointed out: 'I doctor myself, as far as, you know, if it's a cold. . . . I hang on and hang on. Mind you, it's wrong, because you're not fair to the doctor.' On the one hand, then, one 'ought' not to bother the doctor because he's such a busy man; on the other one 'ought' to give him the chance to cure early. Moral imperatives, as we shall see in Chapter 4 on women's and doctors' views on what makes you ill, are all-important.

A 'good' doctor may be both good and bad. The very exercise of power over patients that we object to, in our healthier and more collected moments, may become when we are ill the reassuring expression of omnipotence: it may subordinate us, but it also seems to subordinate our illnesses and anxieties. It is one thing to be brave when we are well, to talk about the importance of assertive patients, of good doctors handing back to the patient the responsibility of her own health. When we are sick, the picture sometimes changes. A woman who spends her life looking after others may occasionally feel the need to become a child again, to be looked after, to have the responsibility for decisions taken away. It is one thing to know in theory how to overcome nervousness when going to the doctor's, or to avoid remembering other things we wanted to ask just after we've closed the door. It is another thing once you are sitting in front of the doctor.

Even if doctors are not omnipotent, if we are ill and afraid it is sometimes nice to believe that they are. Any patient, particularly any mother, knows that there is still a 'magical' element to going to the doctor or calling the doctor. Call a doctor to a sick child, and the chances are she'll be running happily around by the time he arrives. Rehearse the problem that's been bothering you for weeks while you're in the doctor's waiting room, and it will often begin to seem less important before you even go in to the doctor: the pain will subside as you go into his surgery, the rash disappear, the lump in the breast suddenly become impossible to locate.

This magical or symbolic element about going to see the doctor was well recognised by the women we spoke to, and is a central aspect of the power relationship. It is easy to assume that this relationship, as it is an exercise of power, is always and everywhere undesirable. But that is too simple, and we need to take account of the fact that even power may be used in ways both good and bad. What women think of their doctors, the subject-matter of this chapter, is often highly coloured by what doctors 'ought' to be like, and our fantasies of a 'good' doctor. As one patient said to me of her highly competent and thoughtful doctor, a doctor who was also a feminist: 'She doesn'ae seem like a doctor. . . . She doesn'ae even look like a doctor.'

We have seen here the sorts of skills which patients value in a doctor: kindness, listening, time, continuity of care, or the opportunity to get to 'know' your doctor. Potentially, General Practitioners are in a better position to provide this sort of care. In Ann Oakley's study *From Here to Maternity*,[14] Lois Manson complained of the hospital: 'I've not seen the same doctor twice. I mean, they're efficient and what have you. . . . I'm sure I'm a pain as far as that is concerned, but I do think they could be nicer.' About one-third of the women in Oakley's study had shared care between hospital and GP. Reflecting perhaps the more personal approach of the GP, 88 per cent of the women who had shared care would go to their GPs in a future pregnancy. The women in Ann Oakley's sample who had all their ante-natal care at the hospital saw an average of *nine* different doctors, with an average length of consultation of 3.9 minutes.[15] Hardly time for much of the listening valued by patients to take place. Similarly, a recent survey on miscarriage put GPs well to the top of the list of 'helpful' people (with hospital doctors much less often deemed helpful, and sometimes referred to as positively unhelpful).[16] A recent London study evaluating maternity care in general practice found that while 88 per cent of the GP unit deliveries had been 'very happy' with their care, this was true of only 66 per cent of those booked for the consultant unit.[17]

Still, as one of the respondents, added: 'They [GPs] treat you very well, they always call me Mary. . . . But on the other hand, I don't feel I can call him by his first name. You're still a supplicant.'[18] These examples lend some weight to Gail Young's[19] contention that there is potential for change in general practice, and potential (even if not always realised) for less hierarchical relationships between women and their doctors.

Chapter 3

What do doctors think of their women patients?

'Men, I think, tend to be a little more, er, factual. They . . . they'll come in, they'll nail down the points that they want to talk about, one, two, three, whereas women tend to come in a bit vague and then I have to try and fix them . . . pin them down. . . . It's easier from my point of view to talk about a specific worry. I can eliminate a worry about health . . . whether you've got cancer, VD, heart disease, or anything like that. But a women who comes in and says, "Oh dear, I feel fed up, I'm shouting at my husband. . . ." and I say, "Are you worried about anything?" and the answer's, "Oh, no, I've got nothing to worry about," that's what makes it difficult for me, you see.' (GP discussing men and women patients.)

She is an exceedingly healthy looking, cheerful, nicely dressed, good looking woman with a beautiful head of auburn hair without one grey hair in it and she looked at least ten years younger than her age in the manner of a settled neurotic. . . . As you would expect with a neurotic woman, she was frigid, or at least pretty rigid. . . . she has always been full of self pity. . . . I hope that I haven't sounded too critical about this lady in my exposition of the case but it is a fact that after thirty years of looking after these rosy healthy ladies and watching their hair turning more and more auburn when my hair has turned whiter and whiter under the strain of looking after them, I can't help feeling that it is an extraordinary thing that all their

> suffering only results in their looking better and better whilst all my good health only results in my looking a damn sight worse. . . . To get back to a more co-operative attitude towards things, I would say then that she is suffering from a chronic anxiety neurosis with a chronic hypochondriasis, and I would say that she will never wear out. (Letter from a psychiatrist to a General Practitioner.)

The relationship between those providing a service and those being provided with it is often a very complex one. The providers will often feel resentful towards their clients, but their ability to express their resentment either secretly or openly, differs from one job to another. Hotel waiters, it is reported, pee in the soup of difficult customers; shop assistants disgruntled with their conditions of work can take their feelings out on customers by being surly. On the whole, direct forms of action such as these are not open even to the most sorely tried of General Practitioners, though the large number of doctor–patient cartoons emphasises the latent tension in the relationship. When we are looking at women patients, in particular, and predominantly male doctors, there is added tension.

But how much do we know about doctor's views of patients? And where do these views come from? There is rather more data on doctors' views of patients than on patients' views of doctors. While 'how I feel about my doctor' may be part of the patient folklore, and a sentiment frequently discussed with friends and family, it is unlikely to form part of a published or written account. Doctors, on the other hand, do write about their patients, both directly (in medical records and in articles about the doctor–patient relationship) and indirectly (in medical textbooks). This chapter uses some of these data, as well as data from interviews with General Practitioners about their women patients, in order to illustrate the way in which a particular system of values and beliefs about the world structures and influences (often unconsciously) what goes on between doctor and patient. In other words, as some of the examples in this chapter will demonstrate, the General Practitioner tends to offer the patient not only medical treatment, but also a set of social values about what it supposedly means to be a woman. These values are not explicitly presented as such, but are interwoven into the consultation, forming a seamless web.

Most GPs have a list of between 2,000 and 3,000 patients; during their surgeries, they will see from eight to twelve patients an hour (some see many more). However much a doctor may want to treat each patient as an individual, with a workload like that, it is likely that he or she will have some shortcuts for making deductions about patients as they come in the door. Some of these deductions will be biological, some cultural or ideological. Dress, colour of skin, accent – all may indicate something to the doctor. Whatever their scientific training, doctors are no more immune from social or cultural stereotypes than the rest of us. Their social background, education and the advertisements from drug companies which assail them every day may make them particularly susceptible to sex-role stereotyping. Doctors' views on which patients cause them most trouble certainly suggest this, and some light is thrown on this by Gerry Stimson's article 'General Practitioners: Trouble and Types of Patient'.[1] Stimson points out that[2]

> young mothers with families, the insecure, and those away from their relatives are problems for doctors because they are more likely to consult, to come with illness of a type that is difficult for doctors to diagnose and treat, and to have attitudes and behaviour that are not liked by doctors.

Invited by Stimson to describe those patients who caused least and those who caused most trouble to the doctor, General Practitioners made some interesting observations. (There was only one saintly doctor who said that treating his patients was a privilege and that he was therefore not prepared to classify them in terms of trouble.)[3]

In terms of the various social groups into which people could be categorised, men were least, and women most, trouble. In terms of illness, not surprisingly, the healthy were least trouble, as were those with specific organic or physical symptoms, those who were easy to diagnose, treat and manage, and those who got better. Those who presented the opposite characteristics were most trouble, including those with vague symptoms and social problems. In terms of behaviour, the undemanding patient who doesn't consult, who is grateful, co-operative and has confidence is least trouble; the demanding, ungrateful, critical patient is most trouble. In terms of social competence, the patient who is least trouble has a good home, can cope, is intelligent, happy and settled. The unfortunate patient with a low IQ, who is lacking in common sense, who can't cope, and is unhappy and unsettled is most trouble, according to General Practitioners responding to Stimson.

It can be seen from this that the GP quoted at the beginning of this chapter was not atypical. Like the doctors in Stimson's study, the patients he found difficult were women with vague complaints whom he couldn't really help. Since so much of medical training is to do with curing well-defined pathological conditions, it is hardly surprising that faced with a patient whose problems he scarcely comprehends, let alone can do anything about, the doctor feels frustrated and annoyed.

A study of physicians' responses to patients conducted in Canada[4] and published in 1978, confirmed some of Stimson's findings. While there were no definite trends in relation to a patient's age, in relation to sex, there was a trend towards more 'negative' feelings by the doctor. In other words, the women patients evoked more anxiety and frustration on the part of the doctor; the doctor felt less comfortable, and encounters with women patients tended to end on a less satisfactory note. Although the author did not seek a specific explanation for this, he does suggest that 'this could be due to females presenting more problems of living.'

Doctors may be a problem for women. Are women also a problem for doctors? The evidence of these two studies seems to be that they are; that because of the circumstances of their lives, women are more 'troublesome' and 'demanding'. The question is: how well does the average doctor understand the realities of the average patient's life?

Men patients, women patients

The doctors who welcomed us into their practices to do our research and who gave their time to be interviewed themselves are probably not representative of the profession as a whole. Most of them, for instance, were members of the Royal College of General Practitioners (whose membership is around one-third of all GPs), and some had an interest in research themselves. Given that we came into the practices as sociologists, it is likely that they had some sympathy with social problems and social research. In a profession not startling for its radicalism, then, the opinions of these doctors are probably well to the more open-minded end of the profession.

Paradoxically, of the doctors we interviewed, it was almost certainly the doctor who had the most traditional attitudes towards the differences between men and women patients who seemed to have the highest count of 'He's a wonderful doctor' remarks from his patients. He is a kindly, middle-aged male with two teenaged children. His wife is involved in voluntary work, and he runs a single-handed practice on the East Coast. He is a fairly active member of the Royal College of General Practitioners, and normally does his own emergency and out-of-hours work. He was one of the doctors we got to know quite well, since we had carried out some preliminary research in his practice, attended practice meetings together with other staff attached to the practice, and – with the agreement of his patients – sat in on consultations over a period of three weeks. He knew his patients well, and he liked them. They certainly liked him. (On the only occasion when a patient declined to have us sit in on her consultation, it was because she wanted to give the doctor a bottle of whisky as a token of her gratitude to him for helping her.)

He combined a disarming modesty with a highly paternalistic attitude towards his patients. 'My job,' he said, 'is to steer them . . . is to make them as comfortable as possible in life.' He had clear views on the differences in roles between his men and women patients, and the ways in which these might affect the course of an illness. He said of men:

> 'Money is a thing, I think. I think from the male point of view, that people are keen to get back to work because of the money, especially those doing piecework. Anything, anything like that. I'm sure this plays a part.'

This was not so true, apparently , of women:

> 'From the women's point of view, they are anxious about their family, they are anxious about their husband having to do, I am generalising now, I mean, you'll take plenty of examples where this is not true, but taking it by and large, they are loyal to their husbands and they don't like their husbands to have to do the work, look after the house and go out to work. I usually say, "Well, that's his worry, don't worry about him, you get better." But they feel they want to get back to looking after the family. I think the majority of people do, those that don't are usually psychologically unsound, can't cope with the stresses. . . . Not necessarily the screaming abdabs, but, er, being just, being unwell, or developing an anxiety state and . . . or, or sometimes, developing some . . . or making the most, not consciously, of a physical complaint.'

Among the records at this GP's surgery was that of a woman who went very rarely to the doctor's. She declined to be interviewed by us, and in fact had never consulted the GP we were working with. She had, however, consulted his predecessor about fifteen years previously. He had written a curious diagnosis on her card: 'Brainstorm'. She had rarely consulted the doctor prior to this visit, and had not been back since. The correspondence between her GP and the consultant psychiatrist unravelled a rather striking story. According to a copy of a letter the GP had sent to the psychiatrist, this mother of two in her early thirties had woken up one morning and decided that she was fed up with housework, was not going to do any more, and that was that. Her husband (no doubt realising the gravity of the situation) quickly had her down at the doctor's. She did not have any other plans for her life, but she was clear that housework was out as far as she was concerned. Clearly, the problem was immediately defined by all parties involved as a medical problem with a medical solution. One might charitably try to understand the husband's alarm. The wife might well have felt the same way had he woken up one morning and said that he wasn't going to work any more – no other plans, but definitely no more going to work. What was more difficult to understand was that not only did the doctor accept this as a medical rather than, for instance, a social problem, but that he also arranged for her to have a domiciliary visit from the psychiatrist. It was not clear from the correspondence whether a domiciliary visit was arranged because this was considered to be a psychiatric emergency, or whether the GP felt that the psychiatrist might benefit from having a glance at the house, which by now had not been cleaned for a day. But whatever the reason, the woman was sufficiently disturbed to be admitted to the local mental hospital, where she was given a course of six ECT treatments, and discharged 'well' six weeks later. We had no way of knowing whether her subsequent lack of visits to the GP was due to extreme good health, a wariness of the medical profession, or whether, as has been suggested to us, she is now too busy doing housework to go to the doctor's. In this case, husband, wife, doctor and psychiatrist all appear to have agreed that a woman who decides to give up doing the housework has a psychiatric problem, and, in this sense, this particular (though, one hopes, unusual) case is a good illustration of the ideological nature of the consultation. That is, that going to the doctor's may not be just a matter of getting a medical prescription, but also of getting a prescription for the appropriate way to lead your life.

We put an abbreviated version of the story to the GP now in charge of the practice, and asked for his reaction.

Dr: Oh . . . first one would try to find out why. It would necessarily be a fairly lengthy sort of interview. I'd certainly try to find out why this had happened, assuming that everything was going along normally, and then suddenly she stops, and this points to a stress-load over and above which she can't cope. And this is going to be a lengthy business and I think, though, that eventually there might be a psycholo . . . a psychiatric opinion required . . . but I'd certainly try to find out myself so that I could tell the psychiatrist. I'd be interested to know, interested to know why . . . I mean, we all want to stop . . . I mean, I sometimes feel that I am not going to do any more, that I've had enough [laughs]. Stop now, stop the world, I want to get off. But the world doesn't stop, and you don't get off. . . . But this is quite unusual. I wonder who it was? . . . You presumably looked through the rest of the record to find out what had happened to her since. How was it dealt with? Can you remember?

I: Well, she was, she was referred to a psychiatric hospital and she wasn't there terribly long. She was there perhaps a couple of months, and then was discharged and apparently quite happy to go back to the housework and hasn't been in since.

Dr: So it sounds like distress. Sounds like a certain accumulation of stress-overload. The fuse blew.

Within the doctor's own terms, he was acting as a 'good' doctor. He would explore the problem, and possibly seek further help. He would not define it as being outside his province. As the doctor himself pointed out, this was an unusual case. One would not want to suggest that doctors' surgeries are heaving with women refusing to do the housework and being sent for ECT. And one cannot rule out the possibility that this patient was, in fact, suffering from some kind of mental disturbance. But it did seem that a case like this could serve as a sort of litmus paper to test out doctors' reactions to a woman patient coming to the GP with a problem which not only could be defined as non-medical, but could well be defined as not a problem at all (or, at least, not *her* problem). Betty Friedan's work on *The Feminine Mystique*,[5] which portrays so well the 'problem that has no name' – the difficulties and depression faced by housewives – was well known in the late 1970s when we were doing our interviews. None of the doctors we spoke to were unaware of the impact of the women's movement; one was an active feminist. It therefore struck us as significant that although there were some variations in the reactions of the doctors we spoke to about how they would deal with such a patient, and varying degrees of sympathy with the woman (and with her husband), none of the doctors said that he or she would refuse to define such a woman as a problem falling within their province, and almost all said that if they were not able to help her, they would ultimately seek a psychiatric opinion.

The first part of the reaction – refusing to define a problem as outside one's province – raises one set of problems for doctors, and for patients. The second part – defining the problem as a medical one – raises another. It is extremely difficult for a doctor to say to a patient, 'This is not a problem,' or 'This is not a problem which should be brought to a doctor.' Part of the ethos of general practice is that people who consult for inappropriate reasons are not sent elsewhere without at least a hearing. They may eventually be sent to the Housing Office, a social worker, to a marriage guidance counsellor, but they are not told when they arrive at the doctor's, 'You've come to the wrong place.' For the patient, this has the advantage that she or he has a point of access for almost any problem; for the doctor (however much inappropriate consultations may be disliked), it confers an enormously wide sphere of authority. Once a doctor has accepted a problem for discussion in the surgery, all his or her training (to say nothing of daily exposure to drug company advertisements) leads him or her to see the problem in medical terms. (The ways in which doctors can define patients as ill, and patients collude in this, is discussed in more detail in later chapters.)

There are clearly some areas which are more likely than others to be influenced by the doctor's view of what constitutes 'appropriate behaviour'. Emotional, social or psychological disturbance are all more likely than, for instance, a broken leg, to produce a response from the doctor based on his or her own values and beliefs.

One area which has received a good deal of attention in recent years, and in which the doctor's medical judgment may be influenced by other sorts of consideration, is that of Hormone-Replacement Therapy for middle-aged women. Many of the reasons which lead doctors to prescribe HRT are not to do with the purely physiological accompaniments of the menopause, but arise from an assessment of its social consequences. How, in other words, does the menopause affect a woman's ability to get on with her normal life in a relatively untroubled manner? The answers to questions of this kind stem from assumptions about what it is reasonable for women to expect, and about what it is reasonable to expect of women. And any judgments about a woman's normal social function are not in origin primarily medical.

During the time we sat in on his consultations, several patients spoke to Dr L. about menopausal symptoms. At the time, Hormone-Replacement Therapy was getting a good press on the women's pages of newspapers, and several patients edged towards a discussion of this. The doctor only took it up with one woman, however, and we asked if there was any particular reason for this. Given that many doctors refuse to admit that they are influenced by advertisements or representatives from drug firms, Dr L. was particularly frank: 'I suppose to be honest with this particular question, it might have been that hormone therapy had been pushed to the front of my mind by either something I'd read or by a visit of a rep. . . .' Perhaps fortunately for his patients, he had conservative views on the use of HRT, though he was well aware of pressures to prescribe it:

> 'Perhaps this is male chauvinism, but, actually, I feel that I shouldn't interfere with the natural process . . . the person has got to go through these symptoms to get to the next stage, I wouldn't say down, it might be up, but the next stage of their life. Should we interfere by giving them hormone therapy and making them feel better, but not necessarily helping them to the next stage of their life? . . . I tend to go against hormone therapy for this reason. I might be wrong, I might be letting people suffer more than . . . more than they should be, adopting this attitude.'

Although several of the GPs we spoke to felt more inclined to give HRT to women who were in the public eye, or going out to work, this consideration did not affect Dr L.'s prescribing habits. As he put it:

> 'My sole guiding factor would be as to whether they are coping in their present situation, as to whether they are high-powered executives working, you know, or whether it is just the ordinary housewife, you know, managing their house, managing the husband and the children. If either of them couldn't cope, then one's got to offer some line of treatment.'

Dr L. clearly wishes to be of help to his patients (and probably the recognition of this by the patients was why he was so well liked). Medically, he has reservations about the usefulness of Hormone-Replacement Therapy, but ultimately, he is prepared to offer a treatment if he thinks it might help a patient to cope.

Dr W., a middle-aged woman doctor in the north-west took a similar line. She also had some reservations about Hormone-Replacement Therapy, and particularly about the popular publicity it was being given:

> 'There is this *Sunday Times* sort of attitude to what we might call Hormone-Replacement Therapy, if you know what I mean, and that includes that person, whoever she was, who wrote that rather inflammatory book, and, I mean, they advocate going on to hormones more or less *ad infinitum*. Well, I mean, that's perhaps unnecessary. You're going to have to come to the crunch sometime and come off them.'

She did, however, feel that some doctors were too reluctant to prescribe HRT, describing their attitude as:

> Dr: Typical, typical.
> I: What's that typical of?
> Dr: Oh, it's typical of someone who's never had it, you know.
> I: A man?
> Dr: Oh, well, no. [She may have thought this would imply criticism of her male partner.] I suppose you shouldn't say that, really. But I think if someone's getting symptoms that wake them up at night, and they are itching and sore, you know, with vaginitis, and the husband is getting fed up with this because, you know, they . . . they're not sort of co-operating you know, sexually, I don't see why they shouldn't have some sort of treatment.

She felt that some patients were perhaps in more need of HRT than others:

> 'It's very distressing for someone in the public eye, or

someone . . . someone, perhaps, who's a headmistress . . . who suddenly finds that she's streaming with perspiration . . . you know, it's very embarrassing. Everyone knows what it is. . . . It's all right if you're slaving over a hot stove, I suppose you can put up with it. But if people are watching you getting redder and redder.'

In this sense, she is making a judgment on non-medical criteria. In her view, a professional woman is more likely to suffer embarrassment from menopausal symptoms, and so is more likely to be treated. One would not want to suggest that doctors should put social aspects of their patients' lives on one side when deciding on treatment – it is clearly crucial to understand something of the ways in which patients live their lives. But it is also important to articulate the sort of beliefs which underlie the decisions made. Both she and Dr L. felt that the doctor's relationship with women patients was often mediated through the patient's role as mother. The woman's life within the family, and the man's life outside it, were seen to have a fundamental influence on the doctor–patient relationship.

Like almost all the GP's we spoke to, Dr W. was clear about the division of roles between men and women. She herself was married to a doctor and had given up work when her children were small. She was now working part-time and probably saw more of the women in the practice than her male partner. She explained:

'The women come to me and the men tend to go to him. But not altogether . . . not absolutely strictly, you know. I mean, I have my male clientele, and he has his female clientele, but I tend to see . . . the women tend to come to me. . . . It must be . . . it must reflect some attitude they have, or that my hours are more convenient for them, or that I've known them, a lot of them, when they've been pregnant so that they've had sort of nine or ten compulsory visits to me when they are pregnant, which tends to build up a relationship, anyway – you know, willy-nilly. Because it's an emotional sort of time when you're pregnant, anyway. . . . I mean, I'm quite prepared to look at somebody's sort of hernia or, I mean, he [male partner]

> naturally is quite prepared to do sort of vaginal examinations – but they tend, particularly below the waist, they tend to sort of differentiate.'

Dr J. told us something of the men and women in his practice. The men, he felt, mainly had illnesses and worries related to work; the women, illnesses and worries related to the family:

> 'I see women mostly when they're having babies and bringing young children in, and again when they're elderly with high blood pressure, skin problems, digestive and heart trouble. I seldom see young people between 14 and 19. As soon as they get married, they're here – cystitis, husband not as kind as he was when they were courting, general disillusionment. I see twice as many women as men. Men are very different by nature from women. The woman's at home, washing and cooking; the man doesn't do anything but bring home the main wage packet. By nature, she's more involved with the children. But the children grow up, and with the labour-saving devices, there isn't enough for the woman to do at home. I tell them to get out and do something. I don't know what other doctors do, I certainly advise that myself. . . . For women, perhaps 50 per cent of their complaints are psychosomatic; for men, perhaps 30 per cent would have a psychosomatic side to a physical complaint – for instance, a duodenal ulcer.'

Another GP echoed his views:

> 'The woman's aim is to bring up the family, the children grow up, and a woman quite often feels there is no aim: "The old man is out working and I've got nothing more to do, all I've got is the housework and the sink." '

He also discussed psychosomatic illness:

> 'One has to be careful with these people to exclude anything organic. . . . If I feel I'm not getting anywhere, then I'll try a psychiatrist. The problem with the psychiatrist is, they haven't the time . . . they will have one long interview and a series of short interviews and come out with a mass of pills.'

According to this GP, there was really no such thing as a man malingering, since if he feigned disease, it was likely that he would be actually psychologically unbalanced:

> 'They are not malingering, because malingering is feigning disease, mimicking disease, and a person will only do that if they are psychologically unbalanced. I mean, some people would work on with severe arthritis, would work, and do everything. The next person falls apart. . . . This depends on their make up. . . . It must play a part. And it's not their fault. I think I perhaps take an unusual view of humanity. Sometimes, I think in my mind, "Oh, you know, this is a bit much, he could control this," but you can't put it to them. Very oppressive. You are a doctor to administer to the sick. It is not for the doctor to say, "You are sick, you are not sick," to say whether or not you've got a pain. And one has got to minister to them.'

During the course of observing consultations, we had the opportunity of seeing the diagnosis of 'psychosomatic' made in relation to a variety of patients, men and women (though it was never put directly to the patients). One example was particularly interesting, since it underlined the importance of excluding 'genuine' (non-psychosomatic) illness.

A woman came in with symptoms of dizziness and sickness. She claimed to have completely lost her balance, and to find walking unaided extremely difficult. The doctor tested her walking, examined her ears, and conversed generally about her family and her health, after which he advised her to come back in due course if it did not clear up of its own accord. After she left, he commented that Mrs P.'s was a clear case of 'hysterical' illness – in this case, vertigo. She had a history of such complaints and was 'a constant attender' at the surgery. He maintained that she had some basic psychological disturbance which led her to take refuge in ill-health, but that he simply could not understand what it might be as she had 'a doting husband, lovely kids and a nice house'. Six months later, when we raised this case with the doctor again, he felt the same way. He argued that the patient had a basic psychological problem, but that there was no point in seeing a psychiatrist about it as they didn't have time to do anything other than prescribe 'the inevitable bottle of pills'. In the intervening period, however, two things had occurred which might have challenged the doctor's view, since they revealed contradictions in his approach. First, although he had said that he was sure her vertigo was hysterical, she was in fact subsequently found to have Menière's Disease, which does affect the balance and cause dizziness. Second, although he had said that there was no point in her seeing a psychiatrist, she did subsequently enter a psychiatric hospital following an attack of 'hysterical amnesia' after the death of her husband. After a short period of psychotherapy, she was, he observed, looking better than he had seen her for years. It seemed likely to us that this patient was exhausted with the frustration of minding the house and family, and perhaps had certain problems in her personality and relationships which required attention. Hence, she constantly adopted a sick role, with the consequence that when she actually was physically ill, this was not immediately recognised. That she benefited from psychotherapy indicated that she was capable of insight into her situation. Despite these indications that his original approach to her was not adequate, the doctor could not perceive the problem, nor could he analyse her situation in any but the most concrete of terms. ('She has a nice house, lovely children,' and so on.)

Although it seems to me that it is the stereotypes of 'proper' female behaviour which are the most potentially damaging, it would be wrong to say that there are no similar stereotypes for men. The explicit or implicit view held by the doctors we interviewed was that a man's main goal was to work and support his wife and family, and that a woman's was to care for her husband and children. 'From a male point of view, money is the thing. For men, the worry is about work; for women, the worry is about their families.' Dr M., a woman, was particularly concerned about men taking time off work to look after wives or children who were ill:

> 'I'm never happy when I go into a house and find the husband at home looking after the children or his wife . . . their employers don't like it. They don't like them being off if they're not ill. It gives them a bad work record,

and this makes the men anxious. They might say, "I'll look after her, I'll look after the kids, I'll manage, I'll cope," but they're always worrying about their job, you know. . . . A bad work record doesn't stand you in any good stead and they'll have a word with you eventually. . . . When the men are ill, you can give them a sick note and they'll go to bed. The women, you can't put them to bed because they've got the children to look after, unless they're so bad the husband will stay at home. But the husband is the breadwinner, really. . . . But, I mean, practically every family, even if the woman goes out to work, the husband earns the money, really, he earns the most money, you know, and I suppose we haven't quite got to the stage in the culture where men and women are interchangeable in the home, have we?'

The medical textbooks

Another way of seeing doctors' attitudes to their patients is to look at medical textbooks. It is these that provide the written basis for medical training, and which, as in any profession, express and preserve orthodoxies. The view of women and of their illnesses and problems presented in these books does not, of course, determine the conduct of doctors. But it does express the views of the most influencial practitioners of one generation, and influence those of the next. A useful (and much used) book for trainee GPs is *The Future General Practitioner*[6] which gives considerable weight to good communication between doctor and patient. The book presents a generally compassionate approach to general practice, but seems to suffer from the fact that it was written by a working party of six men (helped by one woman committee clerk). Remarkably few of the large number of advisers and critics acknowledged are women (though all twelve of the editorial and secretarial helpers are female). Perhaps the all-male authorship of the book affected both the description and resolution of the following case study:[7]

'A very attractive girl of 19, new to the practice, came for the first time one morning, complaining of tiredness and headaches. She was wearing an exceptionally short skirt, and moved provocatively. Fairly quickly, she revealed a number of resentments. Having been used to a gay single life, she was now tied down both by a small baby and by a very jealous husband. Her husband had recently allowed her to discover that he had been unfaithful. He had also, the previous week, invited a bachelor friend to the house for Saturday evening and Sunday, knowing that the latter found his wife attractive. The evening had been spent watching television, the friend cautiously flirting with the girl. The next morning the husband told her to take breakfast into the other man, and then burst into the room just as the latter was beginning to make sexual advances. The girl resented her husband's outburst about something which had not even happened, especially as he was being actively unfaithful himself. Further questioning revealed that her husband was 12 years older than she was and was convinced that he was very ugly, an opinion which she did not share.

Clearly, the husband had low self-esteem and low security; he felt sure he could not keep his attractive wife unless he tied her down. He tried to bolster his self-esteem by an extra-marital affair; and he set up the situation with his friend both to punish himself and as a further pretext for tying his wife down. The girl had high security based on her proved attractiveness, but her self-esteem had been hurt by the restrictions of her life and her husband's infidelity.

The situation was unravelled with the patient, who began to understand that her own dissatisfaction could be resolved by an occasional flirtation (since she loved her husband), but that his greater needs led him to more extreme actions. She even managed to take this as an oblique compliment (by the husband and the doctor) to her own attractiveness. She left the interview with no prescription and an appointment to return in a week. At the second consultation, she said she felt perfectly well, was getting on very well with her husband, and was not sure what all the fuss was about.'

She still, presumably, had a young baby and a very jealous husband, a doctor who referred to her as a 'girl' and showed an interest in her short skirts. She did, however, have an understanding of the 'greater needs' of her husband which she must now attempt to meet. She may, as the authors say, have left the surgery with no written prescription, but she did leave with a clear prescription of what was expected of a woman in this sort of situation: the needs of a bullying and unfaithful husband who is prepared to use his wife as a sexual pawn must be met and understood. How would the trainee GP have felt if she or he were confronted with a rather different case study: 'A very attractive boy of 19 came to the practice. . . . He was wearing an exceptionally close-fitting pair of jeans, and moved provocatively. . . .'?

In another book for General Practitioners,[8] Dennis Craddock appears to confuse the biological and the social. 'The vast majority of women', he writes, 'have a *basic need* [my emphasis] to have a home and children of their own.' He goes on to describe an 'immature patient' in terms which make the power in the doctor–patient relationship amply clear.[9]

> Mrs A. is a small wiry little women in her fifties, who dresses and acts almost like a teenager. She was the most consistently rude and demanding patient I have ever met, but is gradually beginning to toe the line. She demanded that I should take her blood pressure, and also tell her exactly what it was. 'X used to,' she said when I refused to do this. We seem to be reaching a stage of equilibrium whereby she behaves fairly reasonably and comes to me for reassurance when concerned about her health. Looking back on it, it's been quite fun! The husband incidentally is a pleasant even-tempered chap to whom she is devoted. Had he been otherwise she probably would not have been able to survive outside hospital.

In areas of medicine which affect women only, the prevailing orthodoxies can appear bizarre. Diana Scully and Pauline Bart, in their article 'A Funny Thing Happened to Me on the Way to the Orifice: Women in Gynaecology Textbooks,'[10] looked at the contents of twenty-seven general gynaecology textbooks published since 1943. They divided them into three periods: pre-Kinsey; post-Kinsey and pre-Masters and Johnson; and post Masters and Johnson. The textbooks, say Scully and Bart, 'revealed a persistent bias towards greater concern with the patient's husband than with the patient herself. Women are consistently described as anatomically destined to reproduce, nurture and keep their husbands happy.' In the period 1943–52, of four gynaecology textbooks examined by Scully and Bart, only one presented a strikingly egalitarian approach to sexuality. Two instruct gynaecologists to teach their patients to fake orgasm: 'It is good advice to recommend to the women the advantage of innocent simulation of sex responsiveness, and as a matter of fact, many women in their desire to please their husbands learned the advantage of such innocent deception.' Another advised: 'The fundamental biologic factor in women is the urge of motherhood balanced by the fact that sexual pleasure is entirely secondary or even absent.' Women were assumed in the same text to be 'almost universally generally frigid', while the male 'is created to fertilise as many females as possible and has an infinite appetite and capacity for intercourse.'

Once Kinsey's report had been published, the texts did not ignore the findings. They did, however, use findings which repeated old stereotypes, while ignoring those which challenged conventional views (for instance, Kinsey's finding that, for most females, it was not physiologically possible for the vagina to be the main locus of sensory stimulation). According to Scully and Bart, 'As late as 1965, gynaecology texts were reporting the vagina as the main erogenous zone. The vaginal response continued to be described as "the mature response".' The work of Masters and Johnson similarly left gynaecology textbooks unaffected. Perhaps among the more extraordinary statements quoted are reflections on the sex roles. Scully and Bart quote Jeffcoate, the author of a British textbook: 'An important feature of sex desire in the man is the urge to dominate the woman and subjugate her to his will; in the woman acquiescence to the masterful takes a high place.'[11] A text as late as 1968, quoted by Scully and Bart, suggests of the gynaecologist: 'If like all human beings, he is made in the image of the Almighty, and if he is kind, then his kindness and his concern for his patient may provide her with a glimpse of God's image.' The authors of this article conclude: 'Gynaecologists, our society's official experts on women, think of themselves as the woman's friend. With friends like that, who needs enemies?'

The fact that many gynaecological textbooks are less than fair to women, give a less than accurate picture, and are partial in their use of evidence, does not mean that all gynaecologists have the attitudes implied in the texts above, but simply that it is considered appropriate for the ideological to be presented alongside the factual in a crude, unscientific and patronising way.

Have more recent books now taken such criticisms into account? This was explored by Mary Ann Elston[12] in 1981. Jeffcoate does indeed make reference to changing times in his preface to the 1975 edition of *Principles of Gynaecology*.[13] He writes that he has attempted to preserve the 'personal flavour' of earlier editions and that[14]

> In so doing, I re-stated some of my firmly – and allowing for up-dating from time to time – consistently held views tested by clinical observation and experience. This was against a background of recent developments in knowledge and techniques . . . and in the light of supposed and much advertised, yet probably non-existent, major modifications in the basic outlook and behaviour of the women and girls of western societies.

As Mary Ann Elston points out:[15]

> the 'clinical observation and experience' of doctors is *more* valid than women's observation and experience, even when it is women's experience that is being referred to. This 'clinical experience' is paramount even when unsupported by more systematic evidence such as controlled trials.

Elston did, however, see some change for the better in textbooks published in the 1970s. There are more frequent references to the need to consider womens' feelings in childbirth, though there are few direct responses to the women's movement – apart from that provided, interestingly enough, by our friend Jeffcoate, who writes:[16]

> In the woman, sexual feelings are dormant compared with those of the man, and only develop gradually with experience. . . . Some women never achieve vaginal orgasms and always depend on stimulation of the clitoris, vulva and extra-genital erogenous zones for satisfaction. Indeed, one current view denies the existence of the phenomenon of the vaginal orgasm . . . but most women with satisfactory sex lives have no doubt that vaginal orgasm is real and much more powerful than that induced by superficial stimulation. . . . The above views [i.e. his] long established and confirmed by nearly all normal women are an anathema to small pressure groups agitating for the liberation of women and equality of the sexes in all matters. They protest that the concepts of masculine initiation of sexual activity . . . reflect the prejudice of males in general and of male gynaecologists in particular. And such protagonists maintain that sex drive and desire are spontaneously just as strong in girls and women as they are in boys and men, being motivated by personal pleasure rather than by a procreational instinct or anxiety to satisfy their lover. If this is what they really believe to be true in general, rather than in isolated cases, they deceive themselves, but not others, not even the majority of women. Sex equality in many respects is desirable; but equality in sex desire is unattainable being contrary to an all powerful inherent law of nature.

It is interesting to see just how often 'nature' is used to justify beliefs concerning differences between the sexes. Nature is not always the doctor's friend, however, with 'natural childbirth' often coming in for particular criticism from the professionals. In a piece in the *British Medical Journal* at the end of 1983,[17] an obstetric anaesthetist writes bitterly of wingeing mothers wanting natural childbirth: 'Sometimes it seems that our primagravid patients afford our parous patients the status of professionals, whereas the obstetricians are tolerated as informed amateurs. Advice from the domestic on the ward is to be heeded, that from the obstetric senior house officer disregarded.' Although admitting that 'probably not every woman in labour requires to be managed with high technology' and that 'there is always a grain of truth in every criticism, however emotionally and aggressively made,' the author feels that 'There is currently an obsession among many women about labour and delivery.' Finally, she asks, 'can we not try to defuse all the emotion surrounding the actual birth?'

It could be argued that textbooks on gynaecology dealing with sexual desire are not strictly a part of women's health (though there is a clear prescription in the way that women are treated as *patients*). Similarly, childbirth may be a 'special case' with doctors becoming irked by growing demands from the consumers (the mothers) for a say in what happens in childbirth. And the point should be made that there are, of course, gynaecology textbooks and books and articles on obstetrics which do not objectify the patient, and advocate a respectful and caring stance. What is curious is that there are *any* which do not.

'Thank you for sending me this patient. . . .'

We have seen the way in which some women are portrayed in their records, case notes, and letters from one doctor to another. The lyrical descriptions of women as 'dripping fridges' or references to a psychiatrist's hair getting greyer as his patient's becomes more auburn were mercifully rare. Much more common were references to women patients as 'girls'. The following referred to women aged 55, 48 and 45: 'This girl's cholecystogram is normal'; 'this poor girl'; 'she struck me as being a reasonably level-headed sort of girl.' It is only when we try to imagine male patients of the same age being referred to as 'boys' that we are struck by the full patronising force of mature women being referred to as 'girls'.

Other references were made in notes to husbands of patients, including 'Thank you for sending me this patient, who is the wife of a golfing friend of mine,' and reference to the 'long-suffering' husbands of sick women, particularly those with gynaecological complaints which impaired their sex lives. One consultant physician was visited by his patient's husband:

> Her husband had a long talk to me and has observed that she was able to do the washing up and look after the children at home without too much trouble. He also said that the family situation was deteriorating as a result of his wife's demands for help and attention at home. This confirmed my opinion that a psychiatric opinion may be of value.

Interestingly, it later emerged in an interview with this patient (who was unaware, so far as we know, of her husband's visit to the physician and his complaints about her demands in the home) that at that time, the husband had been having an affair with a women twenty years her junior. The couple were now divorced, but problems had started when the wife had been given a promotion to head teacher – the husband was also a teacher – and had wanted to employ someone to help them (or, as she put it, to help *her*) in the house.

Another consultant physician wrote of a patient, who was admittedly assertive to a point that the unwary consultant might find aggressive: 'Her manner was somewhat unusual.' A colleague to whom she was later referred confirmed this view: 'There is no doubt that this lady is a fairly unusual patient.' Unusual diseases are one thing, unusual patients quite another.

Medical training

Gerry Stimson points out that there are many ways in which doctors develop their views about the nature, problems and illnesses of women: 'there is their medical training, the textbooks they read, their professional journals, and the promotional material sent by drug companies.'[18] There is, in addition, their own social background. Many, perhaps most, still come from social backgrounds where conventional stereotypes of appropriate behaviour for men and women are not challenged, and challenges to these stereotypes will rarely be made at medical school – indeed, there is some reason to suppose that they will be reinforced. Jokes may be made at women's expense in anatomy lectures, comments may be made on a women's physique while she is anaesthetised; students rarely see women in powerful positions in the medical school, but come to see them rather as objects of humour.

There is also some evidence that medical students may actually become less able to communicate with patients as they pass through the medical school. In one medical school, students are given guidance on talking to patients as soon as they enter the school, and a similar exercise takes place in the middle years of their training when their psychiatry attachment starts. A psychiatrist who takes part in both of these courses remarked that the students were *worse* when they attended for the second course than when they attended for the first. The implication was clearly that the intervening period of medical education was, at best, doing nothing to help the way they interacted with patients.[19]

It would be wrong to suggest, however, that doctors' views of patients, of women patients in particular, and of the ways in which they relate to them, have not undergone changes. An influential current has been the Balint School,[20] which has attempted to introduce psychoanalytical insights to general practice. However, although the emphasis on the dynamics of the relationship may well be a useful one, this approach also contains the potential for widening rather than narrowing the gap between a doctor's view of a situation, and a patient's. Stimson and Webb refer to a remark Balint *et al.* make about patients choosing a doctor in a group practice: 'We have found in every one of our research projects that if a patient wanders around in the partnership, this should be considered as meaningful behaviour, that is, as a symptom, which should be properly examined.'[21] As Stimson and Webb point out, such behaviour need not be seen as pathological on the patient's part but 'can quite simply be viewed as an aspect of the strategic behaviour which a patient may use in order to try to get the sort of treatment he wants for a particular problem.' Why is it, they ask, that patients have to use strategies such as this to get what they want? 'Wandering around in the partnership' may indeed be 'meaningful behaviour', but it may mean that it is the doctor, and not the patient, who is unsatisfactory.

Women patients have not necessarily found a friend when they come across a doctor who is really keen on putting her Balint training into action. One Balint-inspired doctor writes:[22]

> One observes not only the words spoken by each patient, but also her appearance and manner, and tries to understand. One not only observes the outward features, mode of dress and grooming, but asks oneself what these may signify in terms of the problem at hand. A patient who adopts a style younger than her years, like 'mutton dressed as lamb' may not do so by accident. She may have difficulty in accepting maturity. Heavy make-up may be a matter of high fashion. It may equally suggest a patient's need to disguise something in herself. A sophisticated or business-like demeanour may reveal anxieties about showing weakness or dependency. A patient who knows it all may be one who has difficulty in admitting her need for help.

One wonders whether any patient escapes from this doctor with merely a kind word and a bottle of cough medicine. It is perhaps fortunate for patients that some doctors feel that they just don't have the time for this kind of approach. As one of the women GPs we spoke to put it:

> 'If you picked up every clue and followed it up, I mean, I would be here twenty-four hours a day. You know you've just got to pick up the ones that you think you can do something about. The situation is absolutely hopeless and you're just going to get yourself bogged down if you follow everything up. I mean, you've just got to pick up the ones you can do something about or else make a mental note that you are going to do it. Sometimes, I do that. I hear somebody say something, and I register it, but I don't follow it up at that moment because it's not suitable. I know there are ninety-five people in the waiting room, you know, but you can always follow it up. I mean, that's one of the things about general practice. You can do it later. Next time they come back, if there's a bit more time, you can follow up what they've said.'

Although things are improving, particularly in the training of General Practitioners, a doctor's traditional training tends to be of little help in (and may actually militate against) the sensitive treatment of patients whose problems are not strictly medical. When facing patients who are clearly finding some difficulty in adjusting to their social situation (the 19-year-old 'girl' with the jealous husband; the woman who was fed up with housework) doctors are in a powerful position to promulgate to their patients a set of social values which are not adequately distinguished from the more 'neutral' medical aspects of the case. Although reinforcing certain social values, the doctors themselves are not creating them, and in many cases, seem barely aware of values and perceptions which structure and influence the consultation. This lack of awareness can be sustained because doctors can often seem to be responding to the views of the patient herself. She will frequently present herself as anxious, dependent, suppliant and inadequate to understand the source of her worries and ill-health. The doctor and the patient then collude together to produce a situation in which the real problems are left undiscussed, and the woman is confirmed in her role as wife and mother. To suggest collusion is potentially 'victim blaming', so the background to this collusion – the way in which it may be internalised as an appropriate, even required form of behaviour on a visit to the doctor's needs some attention and will be discussed in more detail in Chapter 6, 'Making Changes'.

It is, however, precisely this collusion – the expectation or even requirement by the patient that the doctor will behave in certain ways – that makes change so difficult. The doctors who populate this chapter may seem to be a pretty rum bunch, and one needs to reconcile this with the views of the patient. How does the 19-year-old 'girl' feel about her doctor? And what about the woman who didn't want to do any more housework? The chances are that they would not be dissatisfied, disappointed or angry with the doctor. The doctor's 'prescription' (medical or otherwise) may make them feel that there is something wrong with their lives. They are unlikely to think that there is something wrong with the doctor's view of them. This is one of the ways in which the doctor–patient relationship may be characterised by the exercise of power. But it is a power of which patients are not always aware, and one on which they may sometimes depend.

Chapter 4

What makes you ill? Old wives' tales versus old doctors' tales

> 'Sometimes, you gets a bit depressed, but then you looks around the world, you see what goes on, and you thinks, "What you got to moan about?" you know? I never had to go to no doctor.' (Patient who rarely visited the doctor.)

The discussion in this chapter centres on differing ideas concerning good and bad health. A pain may be a pain, an ulcer an ulcer, a cut finger painful, whatever our culture or social group; but we know, too, that illness is part of a whole complex web of social relationships and cultural factors. Even in countries as near each other as Britain and France, for instance, illnesses may be conceptualised in different ways. The average Briton is barely aware that his or her liver exists. The French, on the other hand, are deeply conscious of their livers. An upset stomach, for the English is for the French 'une crise de foie' – literally, a crisis of the liver.

If there are differences of this sort between one national culture and another, are there perhaps differences which are just as sharp beween the views that doctors have on the nature, cause and cures of ill-health, and the views held by their patients? Do women patients, in particular, have different views on the causes and cures of ill-health from those of their (largely) male medical advisers? Ann Oakley and Hilary Graham, looking at doctors' and mothers' different views of pregnancy,[1] argue that they constitute fundamental differences in approach rather than minor variations of opinion.

It seems to me that these fundamental differences characterise almost every relationship beween a doctor and a woman patient. And why should they not? Training to be a doctor and learning to be a patient are very different matters. The picture is slightly complicated, but not greatly changed, by the fact that doctors' views carry an authority which helps to form the views held by women, while the converse is much more rare.

Moreover, given that cultural and social factors are deeply influential in the nature and treatment of illness, it is hardly surprising that those who inhabit such different social worlds as that of the doctor and that of the patient may perceive ill-health in very different ways. All the more so when this is compounded by sex differences. This chapter attempts to show that doctors by no means hold a monopoly on the truth. Or rather, there are doctors' truths and women's truths – doctors' tales and women's tales – which arise from different experiences of the world, different priorities, different evaluations of feeling and doing. It is not a simple division into alternative realities, since, as we shall see, many of the assumptions about what 'being a woman' entails recur in both doctors' and women's accounts of the process of becoming ill.

Though, until very recently, the training of doctors concentrated on the physiological with very little attention given to the psychological, let alone social, aspects of illness, doctors do none the less comment on a woman's illness in terms of her psychological and social situation. Much diagnosis and prescription depends upon a wide range of assumptions about how women ought to behave, what they can reasonably expect out of life, and what function they ought to perform for others. The doctor is always far more than a mere body technician. Yet he or she often brings to the maintenance of conduct an aura of medical scentific objectivity which properly belongs only to the physiological aspects of their work.

But it would be wrong to see this social function of the GP as something which is imposed on unwilling patients. Doctors and patients collude in the medical presentation of social truths. It is probably only a minority of patients who actively resent being viewed, for instance, primarily as mothers or housewives; and in many cases, the process of stereotyping may be so implicit to the consultation that it is not acknowledged in any conscious way by either doctor or patient. However, when such stereotypes affect, or even determine, the advice given to women, it does become a serious matter.

This chapter looks at various myths surrounding health promulgated by either doctors or patients. To begin with, we look at various factors which may be used to 'explain' illness. First, a patient's sex, then age, work, and children leaving home. The idea of 'old wives' tales' (largely a doctors' myth) and 'luck' (largely a patients' one) are then explored together with doctors' and patients' views on drugs and sympathy. This list of social factors whereby doctors may 'explain' ill-health is by no means exhaustive; it could also have included social class, race, or marital status – all areas where there are widely held (mythical) beliefs about the implications for a patient's health. For example, several of the doctors we spoke to had views, not borne out by the evidence, about the relative demands made on GP services by working-class and middle-class patients.[2] Similarly, unmarried women were felt to be a particular problem, although there is some evidence that while marrige tends to be good for the health of men, it has no such protective effect on the health of women.[3] But what of the main focus of this book – the sex of the patient?

The woman patient

Clearly, there are complaints which are related to a patient's sex. It is no myth that some complaints appear more frequently among women than men, others more frequently among men than women. And this does not apply just to reproductive problems. Men are markedly more likely to have treatment for accidents and heart disease; women are more likely to suffer from endocrinal, nutritional and metabolic disease, diseases of the blood and blood-forming organs, and mental disorders.[4] However, much behaviour is falsely ascribed to the biological fact of being a man or a woman (sex) when it should, in fact, be attributed to the social and cultural meanings attached to being a man or woman (gender). Thus, if, as doctors complained in Chapter 3, women tend to come to surgery with 'vague' complaints, this is not necessarily a biological given, but is just as likely to be culturally determined. If men are more likely to make points about what is bothering them, 'one, two, three', this is as likely to be due to their experiences in the world outside the home as to some superior logical ability.

We have already seen that doctors tend to hold particular beliefs about the different 'nature' of men and women patients – beliefs that are largely rooted in social and cultural norms rather than biological givens. To hold these beliefs is one thing. To act on them *as a doctor* is quite another, yet certainly in the use of mood-changing drugs, doctors frequently appear to distinguish between their men and women patients along lines which are suggested by, and presumably not unwelcome to, the drug companies. If a women who lives in a high-rise flat with young children, who is unhappy in her marriage, and who is worried about money can be defined as likely to benefit from pharmacological help, then this is good news for the manufacturers of drugs. (If men, worried about their work, can similarly be categorised, then so much the better.) One story we were told nicely illustrates what may happen if a doctor allows him or herself to be tramlined into ways of thinking based on different conceptions of what men and women are like and how this is likely to affect their health.

A woman went to the doctor suffering from severe migraine. There were many factual statements, both purely medical and predominantly social, which could have been made about her. The ones upon which the doctor concentrated were that she was in her late twenties, a highly successful career woman, attractive and unmarried. Basing his diagnosis on these features of her case, the doctor concluded that the woman's debilitating headaches were due to her social situation – tensions and problems caused by the fact that she was not married, did not have children, was, in short, a 'career woman'. This woman had a twin brother. He also suffered from migraine. For him, however, the facts which were considered relevant to define him as a patient were different, and were medical rather than social. Since his sister suffered from migraine, the cause was undoubtedly genetically determined and biochemical. No social explanation was even attempted with the man. He was not told that he was spending too much time at home with his wife and children and not enough time at the office. He was not told that his headaches were the result of 'overwork'. He was given a biological explanation. Presumably, his sister too could have been told of biochemical changes which caused the headache, but for her, a social explanation was obviously considered more appropriate.

While a patient may be a patient as far as the doctor is concerned, sex does make a difference. It has been shown that fathers bringing a child to the GP's surgery are viewed and treated in a rather different way from mothers undertaking the same task.[5] Perhaps more disturbingly, there is also evidence from a study in the late 1970s that where men and women patients went to the doctor with the same complaint (five complaints were studied) men were given a significantly more extensive physical examination than women.[6]

We talked to the women patients we interviewed about health differences between the sexes. Perhaps leadingly, we asked: 'What do you do when you feel ill? Would you go to the doctor?' These questions were followed by: 'What about your husband? They say that men are less willing to put up with illness than women. What do you think?'

The answers of the patients fell into two distinct groups. The larger group of women said how 'good' their husbands were, how they were never ill, and would rarely go to the doctor: 'Oh, he's good, he never has to go down to the doctor.' On the other hand, a substantial minority felt that their husbands were like big children when they were ill. A bout of influenza for the wife might mean a couple of aspirins and struggling on, often in the face of resentment from husband and children that she was not on top form. For the husband, it would be several days in bed, totally cosseted, children creeping round the house. This wouldn't necessarily mean that he would see a doctor, even though it was not uncommon for a woman to say when asked this question that if her husband was ill, he thought he was a gonner. As one woman put it: 'He will moan and groan, but the first suggestion that he might go and see the doctor and: "There's nothing wrong with me, it's not bad enough to see a doctor." But I can tell that he's not well, so I look after him.'

On the whole, a husband does not need to go to the doctor to 'prove' (at least to his wife) that he is ill. Part of what is understood by being a good wife is noticing when your husband is ill and looking after him. This isn't part of what is understood by being a good husband. Several women felt that they could drop dead before their families would notice. One woman said: 'He'll do the housework if I'm ill, and I mean ill in bed, not just off colour.' Another explained of her husband:

> 'He's very good. He has had to look after the house when I've been in hospital. My mother has looked after the children during the week, but at weekends, he always had them to look after. Mind you, I think it was the last time I came out of hospital – I'd had a hysterectomy – and when we got back home, we came inside and sat down and he said to me: "Oh, please go and make a cup of tea. I've had enough. I feel faint." I think possibly he finds it a strain, but he's quite willing to do it.'

There was little spirit of resentment among the women that their husbands were like babies when they were ill, and yet found it difficult to cope if the wife was sick. Like doctors, most of the women had firmly held beliefs about sex differences in illness. They accepted that they were the stronger sex.

So, on the one hand, women are more likely to have their illnesses treated not as the consequence of some treatable physical cause, but as the inevitable result of being a woman, or, as in the migraine case, of trying to step outside the prevailing (male) view of what being a woman entails. On the other – and the two are aspects of the same phenomenon – women collude in this discrimination, and treat their husbands' illnesses, however sceptically, with far more caring and consideration than they ever receive at home themselves. Women, it seems, can never win. Either they should soldier on, or, if they can't, that probably only proves that they were trying to march in the wrong direction.

It's your age, you know

If the sex of a patient is one factor which helps the doctor make a decision about what is wrong and how to treat it, age comes a close second. A recent letter in a women's magazine goes as follows:

> I was prepared for jokes from my sons and nephews when I had my 50th birthday, but not for the attitude of the medical profession. My sight, my hearing, my teeth, are, it seems, 'not bad for a woman of 50.' They are the same eyes, ears and teeth I had when I was 49.

The stoical humour of women may mask or briefly alleviate the feeling of injustice, but it can never remove it. One patient we spoke to described how she had pre-empted her doctor's questions:

> 'Once, I went to the doctor. I'd got trouble with my back, and the first thing I said was, "Don't ask me my age, because it's not my age." Oh, he did laugh. Because the first thing he always asks is: "How old are you?" And then he says, "It's only to be expected, it's your age you know!" '

We know that ageing in our society has different meanings for men and women. 'An older man' has attractive connotations, perhaps because what he might have lost in looks, he might have gained in money or power. To call someone 'an old woman', on the other hand, is an insult. We have already seen in Chapter 3 the way in which doctors may comment on the differing effects of the ageing process on men and women. Some of the writing on the menopause confirms the view that ageing is supposedly a dreadful process for women. Kalle Achte, a psychiatrist, wrote in 1970:[7]

> The person feels that evening is closing in. Many a woman experiences the cessation of the menstrual cycle as lowering her self-esteem. Fears of loss of youth and beauty occur frequently at this stage of life. Self-esteem and depression are closely related . . . the female feels she loses something of her femininity with the cessation of the menses and she may also be afraid that her sexual partner may forsake her.

A doctor we spoke to had similar views on the disastrous effect of ageing on women, though his experience of its effects on the relative sexuality of men and women was rather different. In his experience:

> 'Men in responsible jobs sometimes need help from anti-anxiety agents. They worry about their responsibilities, and communicate that worry to their wives, and then that ruins their sex lives. Of course, if they're taking drugs for hypertension, that can cause impotence, too. I tell them that, but it doesn't seem to bother them. Oh, but their wives don't like it one little bit.'

Psychiatrist Achte also points out that the diseases that are more likely to afflict women as they age may result in hysterectomy or mastectomy. After such an operation:[8]

> Many physicians certainly know how seriously a woman often takes hysterectomy or mastectomy. She frequently has feelings of inferiority following the operation, as if she were no longer a woman at all. . . . Like the ability to give birth to children, bodily inviolability symbolically means femininity to many a woman, and an excision of the genital organs is experienced as a violent injury. These relationships are often unconscious, but they may also be conscious.

Could such a relationship be unconscious? Would a man, with greater fortitude, view the removal of his penis or testes with equanimity? And is it worry about their femininity which produces 'a proneness to depression' among women who have had a mastectomy or hysterectomy, or is it worry about the fact that they may have a life-threatening illness?

A Family Doctor booklet *So Now You Know About the Change of Life*,[9] bought in a chemist's shop while I was preparing this book (though fortunately now replaced by a much less alarmist booklet), begins encouragingly: 'The Change of Life. The very phrase alone is still sufficient to send a chill shudder through the hearts of many women.'[10] The booklet assumes that '*at this stage in her life*' (my emphasis) the concern of the middle-aged woman should be for her younger relations and friends and that it will give her pleasure to bring happiness and help into their lives: 'This transference of interest from herself to others is the essence of growing old gracefully.'[11]

For most of the women we spoke to, the larger part of their adult lives had been devoted to the interests of others. Far from transferring their interests from self to others at this stage, their 'other-centredness' was often practically built in by middle age. So much so that often, even those who sought other interests, and welcomed this stage in their lives as an opportunity to pursue them, felt constrained from taking them up: 'I'd like to go [to evening classes] but I don't have time. . . . In fact, my husband, when he comes in at night having been away all day, he expects me to be here. I must sit, be around.'

Several women who wrote in to a national newspaper after an article on women and their doctors talked about the relationship of age to health. Mrs S. wrote:

> At the age of 43, all my symptoms of backache, giddiness, light-headedness etc. are 'all part of the privilege of being a woman, so I am excused', I was told 'life beings at 40'. I bet it was a man that thought that one up. . . . My next return ticket to life has already been booked – as a man.

While Mrs J. complained:

> Whenever I go to see my doctor about anything, he tells me that I'm 'paying the price of being a middle aged woman'. I've been to him with backache, headaches and general tiredness. He doesn't investigate at all, but says it is all to do with the change of life. When I was much younger, they blamed all my symptoms on pre-menstrual tension. Next it was because I was on the Pill. Now it is my age. Why do doctors have such off-hand attitudes to women's problems?

Another woman wrote:

> I seldom visit my doctor, but on the occasions that I do, he always asks two questions, how old I am and how many children I have. I tell him twenty six and two and whether I've got flu or backache, he says 'What do you expect?' This happens every time I see him.

Mrs B. wrote how this sort of thing made her feel:

> When I was 50, I went to my doctor. My periods were heavy, I felt weary all the time, kept feeling dizzy and faint. He asked me my age. I told him 50. He replied: 'What do you expect at your age?' He gave me no advice, no medicine, no sympathetic word. I came out of that surgery feeling shattered.

And one patient planned her revenge:

> When I go to my doctor, I can always be sure that he will say 'Oh, it's something doing the rounds' or 'I've just had the same thing myself, dreadful.' I'm longing for the day when I'm pregnant and can ask him whether that is 'just something doing the rounds' and whether he's pregnant too.

On the whole, the women we spoke to, unlike the doctors, did not see ageing as a degenerative disease. Not trained in the heroic mould themselves, they did not seem to expect to need miracles to ease them on their supposedly difficult way through middle age. They were more likely to comment on the degenerative process in their husbands than in themselves. As one of them said: 'Obviously, one does see a great deterioration in men, and I have in my own husband, which of course comes with age, doesn't it? It's something we have to accept.' Another also spoke of the effect of ageing on men: 'In middle age, you realise the world isn't your oyster, and perhaps this affects men more than women, and I dare say this does affect some people and they feel they have to take their last fling – feel that life isn't absolutely first rate.'

Two others specifically linked changes they had seen in their husbands with the sorts of changes that a woman might expect at the time of the menopause. Mrs K. said: 'I think they go a bit moody, just the same as a woman does, only they don't admit it. I think he's ruled by the moon – he can be quite nasty. I think with men, though, it's because they can't admit they're getting older.' While another patient explained: 'I say to him, "I'm sure you're going through the change of life. . . ." I'm sure that they do.' In a third instance, ageing was simply a case of: 'Me husband's not as amiable as he used to be.'

We can see that comments about age are of a piece with the

doctors' views and patients' views that have gone before. The doctors' view is that age is something that they have to bear in mind when looking at the middle-aged woman; the patients' attitude is that what they value is being treated as an individual, and being written off not only as a woman, but also as an older woman, is a double insult.

And do you work? (Only twenty-four hours a day. . . .)

As we have seen, 'work' is a crucial factor in looking at the problems of men and women patients. The doctors with whom we came into contact linked (correctly, in my view) some of the problems of the menopause and of other illnesses of women in their middle years, with stress and overwork. But the solution which they tended to suggest was that women should give up work – meaning paid work outside the home, this being the only category of work they seemed to acknowledge. Our research findings, and the findings of other studies, indicate that symptoms are highest among housewives, followed by those in what can broadly be described as 'working-class' jobs, with those in professional jobs consulting the least. However, it was not the unpaid, and seemingly most stressful, labour within the home that women were advised to give up, but the paid and seemingly less stressful work outside it. This resulted in some curious situations. One woman who did not have paid work outside the home reported:

> 'I've taken on this little girl, and she comes weekends. Weekends, and I have her holiday time. So it's not too bad. . . . And, with the doctor saying I shouldn't work, that it's too much for me, I can't walk any distance and I can't stand any length of time, so it was best, you know, not to work. And we saw it in the paper, they wanted someone to have this little mongol girl, so I applied. It's an interest to me, and, oh, she is lovely. A lovely little girl. What do they call it? Retarded?'

Like the doctor who approved her decision to foster at the same time as suggesting she give up work, she ends up by defining caring for a handicapped child as 'not working'. A psychiatrist took a similar view about a patient referred to him:

> 'I thought that this lady was a woman of good personality who is more than a little stressed because at 54 she has set up house with a divorced man and is trying to do a full-time job and run a big house and satisfy her lover and she is worried about her ability to cope with his children by his first marriage when the divorce comes through. And I think she is a little fraught about whether or not she should marry him when the divorce comes through. . . . I think she should not be at work at this time.'

Such a prescription (along with the prescription she was given for tranquillisers and sleeping tablets) not only places her firmly in her role as housekeeper, lover and potential stepmother, but actually closes off one of her choices for an independent life. Without the independence of an outside job, the decision about whether or not to marry her lover may have become easier, but she is not being helped to make a decision about her life. She is being directed.

Given the social milieu from which most doctors are recruited, and given the views promulgated in paediatric textbooks about the importance of mothers (usually as mothers, rather than as people), it is not surprising that women working outside the home are viewed with about as much enthusiasm by doctors as men working inside it. Those whose experience of domestic labour or looking after children or parents is mainly by proxy may genuinely find it hard to conceive of work in the home as 'real' work, particularly if they themselves live in an environment where an effort is made for all to be quiet on the home front by the time evening surgery is finished. This is perhaps what led Mrs B.'s doctor to make the comment which led her to respond to the newspaper article on women and doctors:

> 'My doctor asked what family I had and what they were doing, and I explained that I have two children under ten and a husband doing shiftwork. The doctor said, "The trouble with you women is you won't put your feet up. It's no wonder you get backache." '

The 'emptying of the nest syndrome'

In so far as the medical profession takes on board the realities of women's lives, a common explanation for distress is that women are unable to cope with their children leaving home – the so-called 'emptying of the nest syndrome'. Within a paradigm where every normal man wants to go out to work to support his wife and family, and will avoid ill-health for that reason, while every normal woman wants to stay at home looking after her children and husband, one can understand the attraction of this 'syndrome', which relies on a whole set of stereotypes about the nature of childcare, household work and motherhood. We know that many women become depressed after having children, and that post-natal depression is so widely recognised that it is a 'normal' part of becoming a mother.

But do most women become depressed at the departure of their children? The women we spoke to didn't seem to think so, although certainly women who have been happy as mothers may feel a pang when their children leave home, and those who have not been so happy may feel sorry that things hadn't worked out as they had hoped, that motherhood wasn't as blissful as they had expected. The one woman who said, 'They can't go quick enough for me,' could not be called typical, but most seemed to find that freedom from responsibility of children had its own compensations. One woman who had had five children and seemed to have enjoyed every minute in spite of living in conditions of considerable hardship, explained: 'We used to have a hell of a time going down the beach, tiddler fishing, going over the hills. And when they was in bed, I got on and done me chores. Now I've got me grandchild, so I still enjoy it. It's better, really. It was hard before.' One woman had heard of the 'emptying of the nest syndrome' and was prepared for it, but it was by no means as bad as she had thought:

> 'Jane's just gone to London, you see, and for a long time I've thought, "This is the last one, I'm going to feel this." There's always been one left, you see. We felt this is an end of an era, when she went, and I admit, I made myself exceedingly busy. But we have more time for each other now, we're free to do things.'

Confirming the view that bringing up children is indeed 'work', several of the women spoke of 'a job well done', of the enormous compensation of seeing their children launched, and perhaps doing well. Josephine T. admitted: 'I was happy for them. . . . I was happy to think that they'd both . . . this sounds awful . . . they'd both found young men of whom I approved.'

Others had occasionally found that the delightful young things who had been their babies and happy toddlers had grown up into teenagers and adults they were by no means so happy about. The dear little piglets had become pigs. As one woman put it: 'They're nicer when they're younger. They need you when they're younger. They need you in a nice way, a very loving way. Now it's, "Mum, can you lend us a couple of quid?" "Mum, will you do this, will you do that for us?" '

It is perhaps not surprising that it was a middle-aged woman GP who seemed most aware of the complexities of children leaving home, even if she showed some of the 'toughness' which women patients claimed to experience from their women doctors:

> 'Sometimes, you do find middle-aged women who fuss, fuss, fuss on about their children as if they were 6 and 7 when they're not, you know. I mean, they are great lads of 16 and 17 – quite capable of opening a tin of baked beans and opening the front door, you know. . . . But, I mean, this is the women who don't go out to work probably. . . . I think sometimes people do miss their children terribly, but then sometimes they don't; after all, it's inevitable. Strangely enough I had two middle-aged women in here in one morning. They didn't know each other, and they both were crying and depressed because their sons who'd lived at home with their mothers were both getting married, and they said, "I'm delighted he's getting married, you know," and wiped the tears away. "But I'm terrified I shall let him down at the wedding, and I shall cry at the wedding, I shall miss him. . . ." They both spoke identically, which was funny, you know, they didn't know each other, and yet they were delighted. You see, people are delighted when their children go to university, delighted they're going to

training college. I mean, perhaps not so delighted they're in prison or something, but delighted if they're doing well. You see, it isn't acceptable, really, for them to grieve over the fact that their children have gone, because it's acceptable that they should go. . . . This is really when they should have made preparations for this before, because it is very difficult to get into something at 45 when you're not skilled. They should get themselves dug into a job they can do at 30. At 45, you're in the very worst bit of the market, aren't you? You haven't got very long to go, and yet actually, you see, people who've worked for a long time and reached 45 are good workers. I mean, they are sensible, they've got a good sickness record, they haven't got to be off because the children are ill. . . . People who do have women working for them who are 45 and 50 and 55 say that they are very reliable, sensible and not hysterical, and they don't have to keep dashing off when the children have measles.'

But if there were sometimes problems about children leaving home, this doctor did not define patients by this fact:

'You get people who are just menopausal . . . it doesn't necessarily mean that you're missing your children or anything. There are plenty of women who've got no problems who have hot flushes, and they want something to ease them. It's jolly uncomfortable.'

As we've seen before, many doctors have a deeply stereotyped view of women and their 'psychology' which may well interfere with their medical judgment. Women may be defined as mothers in such a way that there is no real understanding of the work (as well as the responsibility) involved in being a mother. And even if a doctor recognises the need to take social factors into account, he or she may have little conception of what it means to be a mother, a factory worker, or a single parent (i.e. 'social' understanding can be as stereotyped as 'psychological'). The responsible doctor is, however, aware that there is a problem here. The patient who comes to the doctor with vague anxieties and aches and pains, with problems which appear to have no physiological basis, still needs some help. The potential of the doctor to help in any direct way with problems of poverty, housing, family violence or the depression of a life not totally fulfilled, is limited. Fully aware of the pressure on the General Practitioner (and his or her own wish) to be of help, are the pharmaceutical companies. This chapter is concerned with both causes of, and cures for, ill-health. Drugs fall nicely into both categories.

A pill for every ill. . . .

Coming away with a prescription is so much a part of a visit to the doctor's that, in many practices, part of the receptionist's preparation for each surgery is to write the name and address of each patient attending at the top of a prescription and attach it to the patient's notes. By the end of the surgery, few of these will be unused. And it is not simply the doctors who expect to dispense drugs; it is something that the patient expects from the consultation. A prescription 'proves' you were right to go to the doctor. So deeply entrenched is this idea that many of the doctors' surgeries we visted displayed a DHSS poster asking patients not to feel too upset if they left the surgery 'empty-handed'.

And well might the DHSS worry. Looking at psychotropic drugs alone, during the period 1965–70 non-barbiturate hypnotic prescriptions (mainly sleeping pills) increased by 145 per cent, tranquillisers by 59 per cent and anti-depressants by 83 per cent.[12] Doctors have considerable freedom to prescribe drugs. Given the pressure on them by drug companies and patients, it is hardly surprising that they exercise this ability. But it is not just pressure that leads them to prescribe. All their training leads doctors to expect to be active in the management of the patient and not merely to lie in wait for things to improve or otherwise. One of the ways to be active is to prescribe, and it is also something around which the consultation can be built. Examination of the patient, prescription, explanation of how to take the drug, perhaps some explanation of what the drug is and how it is likely to affect the course of the illness, goodbye as the prescription is handed over – and the transaction completed. Without the prescription, how is the consultation to be constructed?

This section deals with only one small part of the armoury of drugs – the psychotropic drugs. This is partly because there is a wide and significant difference between the number of psychotropic drugs prescribed for women and the number prescribed for men, and partly because the indications for their use are often as 'vague' as the symptoms which doctors claim their women patients present them with. Are they simply vague remedies for vague ills? Are they more useful to the doctor than to the patient? (That they are extremely useful to the shareholders of the drug companies goes without saying.) There are, of course, very large numbers of people for whom such drugs undoubtedly have a marked therapeutic effect. There are large numbers of others where not only is the therapeutic effect in doubt, but where the drugs, by creating dependence, may actually be preventing a full return to health.

In a study published in 1971,[13] Parish found that of 13,259 records examined in detail, 1,668 patients had been prescribed psychotropic drugs during the period of the survey. A large proportion of these were apparently repeat prescriptions. Parish refers to a survey of doctor–contacts and repeat prescriptions which found that one in four patients gets 'nothing' from a doctor except a repeat of a previous prescription. If the drug treatment were continued longer than six weeks, then it was likely to continue further for more than a year. Many patients receive repeat prescriptions without even seeing the doctor. Looking at those groups most likely to be using psychotropic drugs, Parish asks:[14]

> Why are twice as many women as men prescribed psychotropic drugs? What leads so many women to seek treatment for obesity from their general practitioner: what do they expect from him and why does he prescribe appetite suppressants? And what factors lead so many elderly women to attend their general practitioner for the treatment of insomnia? Why do general practitioners prescribe so many hypnotic drugs?

Explaining one of the ways in which psychotropic drugs may be overused, this very clear-sighted and soundly researched report points out:[15]

> Insomnia can be a symptom of mental, physical or social stress and as such, should only be regarded as a symptom of a disorder requiring a holistic approach, so that ideally hypnotics should be prescribed only as short term adjuncts to more specific therapy. As a 'mental' symptom, insomnia must be treated as one of a cluster of symptoms caused by a mental disorder (e.g. endogenous depression), particularly if it is of recent onset and occurs in the absence of a crisis. As a 'physical' symptom it is often secondary to pain caused by some physical disorder, particularly osteoarthritis and rheumatoid arthritis which then should be treated more specifically. Insomnia due to 'social stress' needs symptomatic therapy with hypnotics only for a few nights to help tide the patient over the worst period. Beyond this, it is essential to make more searching enquiry into the patient's problems and symptoms. In the lifelong 'inadequate' personality who repeatedly requires a 'crutch' to help him through life's stresses there usually is little need for hypnotic drugs which are contra-indicated in this group because of the risk of drug dependency. Such patients require superficial psychotherapy and support with only occasional 'sedatives' to help them over acute periods of stress.

In other words, whatever the reason you are suffering from insomnia, there is better treatment than sleeping pills, at least in the long term.

Among the doctors we spoke to, there were those who prescribed relatively large amounts of psychotropic drugs to men and women, and those who did not. It is hardly a world-shattering finding that those in inner-city practices were more likely to prescribe these drugs than those in the country. Partly, it may have been that there were less of the sorts of stresses that called for drug treatment in the country; just as important, though, the rural doctor also tended to have more time to counsel the patient.

One case of a woman who had been taking 5mg of Librium a day (a small dose) for some years is of particular interest. This was the patient in Chapter 2 whose agoraphobia had led her doctor's partner to suggest a stay in a mental hospital if she did not pull herself together. She was a working-class woman. She had three grown up children of whom one, a 30-year-old son, lived at home. She also had a son of 16. Her husband and her elder son were both on shiftwork, but working different shifts ('Like a full-time job for me,' she explained wearily). She tried to explain the process of becoming agoraphobic:

> 'Well, I don't know why it is exactly, although I often sit down and think about it. I know part of it. My father was very ill, it was just before he died, and I was down there on my bike four times a day. And I had this brother who lived with him who was blind and stone deaf in one ear, and they was quarrelling all the time. And in the end, I got off me bike one day when I got home and I thought, "I can't stand it." And after that, I couldn't go out. I couldn't. Not even as far as the gate. But they've both been gone for years now and I'm still the same. I don't know why it is. . . . I can go shopping with a neighbour, and my husband's very good. But what I'd do if he passed away, I don't know. The boy's good, too. It was just before he was born that it came on, or just before I fell for him. We were thinking about having another one, my husband and me, because I was a bit lonely and the kids were growing up, and we went to see the doctor because we wondered if we was too old. Anyway, he looks at my records, because he was one of these stand-ins, because I'd already been with my nerves, see, and he said, "Having a baby, it's the best thing you can do." Well, I didn't know at the time, but I'd already fallen anyway. The boy's always been really good about the agoraphobia, because it must be embarrassing for him, at school and that. He seems to understand. Even when he was little, he seemed to understand. But some people, they think you're barmy.'

I was not in a position to judge whether this woman's problems were, in Parish's terms, 'mental' or 'social'. (Even I could see that they were not physical, except in so far as they may have been related to fatigue.) What was clear was that this intelligent woman had the insight to explore the roots of her difficulties, a way out of her problems (not necessarily a solution) which would have been less costly and less time-consuming for herself and her family, her doctor and the state, than the little mountain of Librium she had consumed.

The drug companies play a big part in the number of tranquillisers taken by women. Stimson looked at a series of advertisements for psychotropic drugs[16] and found that women were portrayed fifteen times as often as men. He writes:[17]

> Women's role problems are defined in medical terms. Beside a pile of dirty dishes, magnified to twice her size, stands a woman with her head resting on one raised hand; in the other hand is a tea towel. Above the picture is the line "When the mind magnifies . . ." and below ". . . Integrin restores the perspective." . . . The advertisements with women also depict the "neglected generation" of older women whose children have grown up and left, the spinster, and the widow. Women's problems seem to be defined mostly in terms of the presence or absence of a husband or children. Those who have a husband and children are unhappy because of the problems of being a housewife. Those who do not have a husband and children are unhappy because they do not have them.

For the drug companies to identify problems in a woman's social role is one thing; to suggest that drugs are what is needed is quite another. Not that men are not also portrayed as needful of medication – this time, to protect them from the world of work. Stimson describes an advertisement showing a middle-aged man behind his desk. The advertising copy goes as follows:[18]

> Behind the calm confident front of the successful management man, nagging doubts are sometimes just discernible. Aware that younger men are coming up, he suddenly behaves irrationally. Or his opposition to some new technique or system is marked by uncharacteristic vehemence, pin-pointing ill-concealed emotional under-

> currents. Somatic complaints are often the first indication that all is not well, the eventual visit to the doctor being prompted by insomnia, rash, headache or other presenting symptoms rather than their cause: anxiety or depression. But this is quickly revealed in consultation.

Elsewhere in his work on these drugs, Stimson points out that drug companies indicate how the doctor can make an 'at a glance' diagnosis. Ever vigilant to the way a woman is presenting herself, the doctor is told by the drug company to look out for symptoms of depression – 'Some attempt at make up', 'respectable façade – i.e. hat, handbag, gloves and even necklace', 'ill-fitting stockings, outmoded lipstick poorly applied.'[19] As Stimson suggests, even if the doctors who are bombarded daily with these sorts of advertisements were not directly affected (in the sense that they did not think: 'Ah, depressed woman this or that particular drug') there can be little doubt that their overall impression of women as patients must be affected by the limited and limiting view of women as presented by the advertisements.

Just as some of the doctors we spoke to were relatively high prescribers of psychotropic drugs and some relatively low, some of the patients, particularly among those who went to the doctor a lot, were high users of such drugs, some of them, who went infrequently, low users. Not surprisingly, the low users were far more likely to comment unfavourably on the use of drugs of this sort. As one of them put it:

> 'I don't really believe in taking things. I think your body has its own resistance, and you weaken it by taking medicines. I might take something for a day or two, but usually, I prefer not to. These tranquillisers, I think they do something to you. They might make you feel a bit better, but they make you dopey. I tried one once, but I felt awful. I thought, "I'd rather think about my problems and know what they are than feel like that" – as if I wasn't myself, you know. But I have friends who take them all the time. I tell them they shouldn't.'

Those who took tranquillisers were just as wholeheartedly in favour of drugs. ('Oh, I couldn't cope without them . . .'). But patients, doctors and drug companies are well aware that there are few situations where pills actually solve problems.

To suggest that many, perhaps most, doctors and certainly most of those we spoke to were not aware of the problems of prescribing drugs of this sort would be unfair. Some spoke openly of their reluctance to prescribe drugs to alleviate social ills (except perhaps on a very short-term basis), but felt that the alternatives open to them were not really satisfactory. Time was the problem. There was no time to spend discussing problems in detail and counselling patients, because of all the other patients waiting to be seen. Meanwhile, the advertising of the drug companies suggests that drugs put patients' problems into proper perspective, and thus make them better able to deal with them themselves. But how much real help is it to a woman faced with a twenty-foot lion to be shown that the beast is actually only ten-feet long? It would be more use to give her a shotgun. In so far as the social and emotional problems which women face are dealt with wholly or in part by drug therapy, the situations which oppress them are maintained by default, and frequently are actually legitimised. There are times when the problems may indeed lie in the woman's consciousness, but there are many others when her consciousness consists of an accurate awareness of a real and oppressive situation in which she, categorised as a woman, finds herself – in the home, at work, in the doctor's surgery.

The importance of sympathy

One area where we found a gulf between doctors' views and patients' views was on the subject of sympathy. Perhaps it is not surprising that doctors, trained in the heroic mode where the 'cure' is all-important, see sympathy as a last resort. It is, perhaps, a sign of a rare humility that doctors do not seem to realise that a few words of sympathy, a murmur of agreement, an acknowledgment that a patient is having a tough time managing, may make a good deal of difference to the way that someone feels. Medical texts I looked at dealing with the problems of middle-aged women tend to deride the idea of treating menopausal women with 'mere' sympathy, or make a distinction between 'genuine' symptoms, which can be treated medically, and 'vague' symptoms, which call for short shrift. The idea that appears to underlie this is that 'real' symptoms are the ones that can be cured. If it can't be treated, it isn't a symptom. If it doesn't fall into place as part of the history of an illness, it's 'vague'. As one text puts it: 'Vague symptomatology, often the result of awareness that the age of forty has been passed and that "change of life" troubles must be expected, does not warrant special treatment.'

This was not the view of the woman who wrote the following:

> If men had half the troubles some women have, something would certainly be done about it. . . . I never gave the change a second thought. . . . I've always led an interesting life. . . . I never dreamt I would be reduced to such depression, lying about just crying, no energy, palpitations, dreadful headaches, waking up wet with sweats, not wanting to meet people and all I've had is valium and 'try to socialise more.' We are not being like this for sympathy because we don't get any. I'd rather be out enjoying myself.

Though sympathy might seem a rather weak solution to the doctor, we have seen that patients think otherwise: 'You can talk, and he'll listen,' 'He's tolerant, very tolerant,' and 'I can talk to him, he's more or less the same age as me,' were among the highest attributes of a 'good' doctor. The 'good' doctor is required both to 'know' and to be ready to learn. He or she must be able both to express understanding of the patient's description, and to wait patiently while it is given. It is not an easy combination, because it involves both the exercise of authority and the performance of a service. Too often, doctors both diagnose over the heads of their patients, and discount what they have to say. They do so especially if what the patient has to say appears to constitute a rival 'truth'. It is for this reason that there is such hostility in the medical profession to the collective wisdom of women patients, and that it is dismissively referred to as 'old wives' tales'.

Luck and the moral concept of good and bad health

The term 'old wives' tales' is, at its broadest, simply a dismissal of the beliefs of women patients. Prominent amongst these beliefs are two views of health commonly found amongst women. Yet though they so often accompany one another, they seem at first sight to rest on quite different systems of values. On the one hand, there is the idea that good or bad health is a matter of luck; on the other, the view that there is virtue in putting up with things, and that people who go frequently to the doctor's, even if genuinely ill, are somehow acting reprehensibly. The one seems to remove all responsibility from the patient for the state of her health; the other to place on her an almost stoical moral burden. Asked how their health had been over the past year and over the past five years, a very general question, women in good health would very frequently 'touch wood':

> 'Touch wood, I've always been, I think in all my life, since I got married, I had one day when I went to bed and I couldn't get up 'cause every time I stood up, I was sick. So that lasted one day, and my eldest daughter was about 11 or 12 and she coped. The only time I've ever been in bed was when I had the kiddies. Touch wood.'

And: 'Touch wood, I feel fine, really, but I did have this slight accident – the burn.' Another, asked what she did when she felt ill, explained: 'I look after myself, well, for a cold or 'flu. But, touch wood, I've never really had anything.' Another woman had had a hysterectomy four years previously: 'But touch wood, I was lovely after that.'

Is it a sign that women don't feel in control of their health that 'touch wood' is mentioned in relation to good health? Is health really perceived so much as a matter of luck, or are the words 'touch wood' a matter of habit rather than a matter of belief? Certainly, we did not find the idea of luck in relation to good health among the doctors in anything like such a strong form. One or two mentioned the element of luck, or the element of chance, some families were characterised as having had 'bad luck' in the way of health. With the doctors, though, the reference to luck was almost certainly a turn of phrase. Ideas of luck fit uneasily alongside the rationale of science. If patients were ill, the workplace might be to blame (though rarely if it were somewhere as unthreatening as the home); smoking, alcohol, or stress might equally be invoked. But luck was alien to the medical view of things. Why did it play a more important role for women? To talk of luck is to recognise one's helplessness. And yet it is also a hopeful belief, with more optimism in it than a belief in fate. Women may not be in charge of their own health, but at least when they talk of luck, they deny that anyone else necessarily has to be either.

Ideas of luck involve a quiet but subversive rejection of the rationale of science. But notions of 'good' and 'bad' patient, often used by the very same people who bring 'touch wood' into play, have a different moral flavour. For many patients, 'I'm very good' or 'He's very good' could be translated as: 'I'm hardly ever ill,' 'He's hardly ever ill. We hardly ever go to the doctor's.' While a sick patient, or one who spent a good deal of time at the doctor's would not characterise herself as 'bad', it was not uncommon for other patients – whether or not they went often to the doctor themselves – to harbour an indignant feeling that there was something 'wrong' about the patients who crowded doctors' surgeries, who consulted with trivial complaints, who wasted the doctor's time. It would be a matter of some pride not to go to the doctor, however dire the illness, to be aware, as we have seen in Chapter 2, that to visit the doctor is to 'bother' the doctor, that the doctor is 'a busy man' and that the 'right' thing to do is to look after oneself for as long as possible, without leaving it so long that the doctor doesn't have a chance to cure you. Those who have the good fortune of health also have the good fortune to be characterised as good: 'Oh, my mother was very good. She was never at the doctor's, never. I can't remember her ever going. Not until a few years before she died and she got glaucoma, but that was all.' It was clearly a matter of some pride to Mrs A. that she hadn't been to the doctor's, even when she was quite ill: 'I try and look after meself. I didn't even go when I had yellow jaundice.' A woman who rarely attended surgery showed that she knew how to use the doctor, and when not to bother him when she said: 'I wouldn't go to the doctor for just any paltry reason at all – I usually doctor myself – take a couple of anadins.' While a woman who spent a good deal of time at the doctor's expressed much the same sort of sentiments: 'I only go down when I've run out of my prescription. I don't bother him for the least little discomfort. I'm like a chemist's shop. I don't need to have to go bothering the doctor.'

But is there perhaps more to this than a deferential wish not to 'bother the doctor'? While there is a desire to avoid intruding on professional time, there is also an assumption of personal competence over one's own health and one's own body. To be able to keep away from the doctor, one has also to believe that one doesn't always need to consult him or her. Women have their own skills, their own little corners and reservoirs of power.

The use made by women of the idea of 'luck' may at first suggest a belief that health is something completely outside a woman's own control. But it implies an equally clear shift of acknowledged power away from the medical professionals. And if luck places good and bad health in the middle ground between doctor and patient, the idea of the 'good' patient seems to place some power, at least, in the hands of the patient herself. If it is up to her to conduct herself properly, it is clearly also in her power to do so.

Old wives' tales

If something is worth attacking, it is usually because it is seen as threatening. The hostility of the professionals to 'old wives' tales' arises in part from a recognition of a rival account of the truth or at least of parts of it. It is not simply that women's own accounts and experiences are regarded as heresies. The professionals sometimes also recognise that women have their own unique skills and insights arising from personal experience. It is their health, both good and bad, which doctors, however skilled and sympathetic can only ever approach from outside: it is their menopause, their childbirth. Women are not observers, but participants.

Particularly in writing for the lay audience, therefore, doctors tend to stress what they see as the 'dangers' of talking to other women. Ante-natal booklets tell us not to listen to 'old wives' tales' – as we have already seen in Chapter 2, a book on the menopause urges: 'She should be chary of talking overmuch to her friends.' This is preceded by the friendly advice: 'She may relate her feelings, and if she has them, dreams, to her doctor frankly and without shame.'[20] However, few old wives' tales paint as alarmist a picture as some medical writing, for example, on the menopause. 'Evening is closing in . . . fears of loss of youth and beauty . . . losing something of her femininity . . . fears her sexual partner may forsake her.'[21] Elsewhere, we find the following:[22]

> At the menopause, the female becomes conscious of the crisis of middle age; she becomes painfully aware that youth is gone and that the remaining life-time is limited. The pain is increased and aggravated by the cessation of the menstrual cycle, which is experienced by many a woman as a diminution in her femininity and self-esteem, and this makes her increasingly prone to depression. The menopausal crisis is, to a large extent, a crisis of human existence; it means that something valuable must be abandonded. Adjustment to the new state of affairs is a time-consuming process, and that which is ahead is being feared.

There can be few old wives' tales more potentially worrying than these respectable texts.

On the whole, the women we spoke to valued talking to other women about their experiences, and valued knowing that they were in the same boat as other women. What is more, in every case where we were told of advice given by mothers, sisters or friends, it was considerably less alarmist than the statements made above. Women patients did not adopt a 'doom and gloom' approach. As the woman whose words opened this chapter pointed out when asked about the menopause:

> 'Well, I've finished now. I haven't seen [a period] for about four years, and to tell you the truth, I haven't noticed anything. Sometimes, you gets a bit depressed, but then, you looks around the world, you sees what goes on, and you thinks, "What you got to moan about?" You know?'

I am not suggesting that there are no women who pass on upsetting stories; but then, some of the things they are talking about *are* upsetting – for example, the ways in which they have been treated by doctors. But on balance, talking to other women is helpful to women, women are a genuine and often under-used resource for good advice, and doctors could well learn from listening a little more closely to old wives' tales.

What this chapter has tried to show is that, particularly as far as non-medical factors are concerned, doctors by no means hold a monopoly on the truth. Or rather, there are doctors' truths and women's truths, which arise from different experiences of the world, different priorities, different evaluations of feeling and doing. It is not a simple division into alternative realities, for many of the assumptions about what 'being a women' entails recur in both doctors' and women's accounts. But much of the understanding about the social fact of being female which informs the actions – and inactions – of doctors, functions to maintain women in particular roles, and exclude them from others. And at the same time, it is contradicted by the 'tales' which women tell each other. The two 'truths' may not always be mutually exclusive, but they often contain antagonistic accounts of the world, and antagonistic values. What, after all, is so wrong about being either 'old' or a 'wife' in the context of 'old wives' tales'? The implied disqualifications are as illuminating as the dismissal of the tales of experience which they express.

Chapter 5

Family matters

Yesterday I went
to the grocery store
I had filled up
the cart
and was half way through
the check stand
before I realised
I had shopped for the whole family.
The last child left
two years ago.
I don't know what
got into
me.
I was too embarrassed
to take things back
so I spent the week cooking
casseroles.
I feel like one of those
eternal motion machines
designed for an
obsolete task
that just keeps on
running.
I certainly don't want them
back either.

When the
last baby stopped getting
up at
night, I didn't stop. . . .
And William never
understood. To him
if you are tired, you sleep.
I have never been able to
penetrate the
simplicity of his logic
which is
after all
the logic
of most of the world.[1]

Susan Griffin, *Voices*

Whatever differences there may be between women in terms of wealth and status, there are clear cultural ideas concerning what it is to be a mum or a wife in terms of caring and nurturing. However much we are told that men and women are taking on similar tasks within the home, more is still expected of a 'mum' than of a 'parent'; more of a wife than of a husband. For whatever a woman's life may be outside the home, the assumption is that her main duties remain inside it, caring and nurturing. But this work within the family is rarely recognised for what it is, either in terms of the demands it makes on a woman's time or on her own health.

Each family has its own pattern of using the doctor, and develops traditions concerning health care, in which mothers in particular will be influential. One woman told us: 'I try not to bother the doctor. I've just grown up with that. My mother always used to dope us up.' Another spoke of the indirect influence of her mother-in-law:

> 'If there's anything on the television about health, my husband makes me turn it off. He says, "That's not entertainment." And he won't let me have a medical book in the house either. I think it's because his mother had a whole lot of home doctor books and was always going on.'

The family is the context within which both good health is produced and poor health suffered. Women within the family recognise both their own roles as producers of good health and also – though less explicitly – the effect that the family may have on their own health. Well under one-third of all episodes of illness come to the attention of a doctor, and by the time they come to a doctor, almost 90 per cent of patients will have had advice or treatment from friends, relatives or chemists.[2] As the textbook *The Future General Practitioner* makes clear, illness in the household creates a disturbance.[3] Something of this was evident in an episode in the previous chapter – the husband who needed a cup of tea when his wife returned from hospital after a hysterectomy, the wife who needed to be sick in bed before anyone else in the house would lift a finger.

Good health may be provided by the mother/wife in terms wider than those of good nutrition and good general care for those in her charge. It may occasionally be literally a 'gift'. Mrs H., the patient whose story started this book, and who commented on the change of attitude in her gynaecologist when she saw him privately, saw this as the sort of medical service she would like her daughter-in-law to have:

> 'It's not right I suppose, but, oh, he was nice. So when my daughter-in-law wanted to go because they wanted to start a kiddie and they didn't seem to be able to, I said to her, "Let us treat you, and you can go on the private." And she had her operation done on the private, too.'

As we see from this, not all the knowledge that women pass on about medicine consists of 'old wives' tales'. There is a concrete material basis here for what is on offer. Mrs. H. had built her life around her family, and she and her GP agreed that moving to the suburbs from the home where she had brought up her family had been a cause of considerable emotional turmoil:

> 'Last Easter, I had an awful depression. I could have done with Freddie [grown-up son] at home then. Well, I went to see the doctor and he said, "I've been expecting you." And I said, "Oh, why?" And he said, "Ever since you moved, I've been expecting you. You've got a lovely house out

there, but you're isolated. When you lived down this way, if you felt a bit low, you probably didn't realise it because you'd pop round Marks and Spencers and buy yourself something to cheer you up. But you can't now, living right out there." Anyway, he said, "Well, you know what happens if you don't fight it, it just comes back again and again." So he said, "You've got to fight it, and you'll win through." He gave me some tablets. I think they were to calm me down a bit. Since then, I've felt I'd like to do a little bit more, maybe a voluntary hospital job. But my husband doesn't want me to. He doesn't object, but he doesn't think my health is up to it, what with that and the housework and me looking after him.'

This patient was not untypical of those we interviewed. She was still living in the town where she had been born, and had married at the age of 20. She had left school at 14 to do shop work, and had then been a typist. She had given up work outside the home when she got married, and had had her first child shortly afterwards. She had three grown-up children, two girls, now married and both of whom had moved away, and a son, also married, who lived locally. I asked about housework:

'Well, it doesn't take much time now I've got all these labour-saving gadgets. This house is no trouble at all. When we moved here, he bought me an automatic washing machine, so I don't have a day for washing any more, and a tumbler drier, so I can even do the washing if it's raining. We can have clean sheets twice a week now.'

Did her husband and children ever do housework?

'Well, the girls helped. The windows is all my husband would do. He's not one of those domesticated men. I'm a golf widow and a football widow. I like to think he goes out. Probably his work is harder than mine is. . . . I'm glad to get rid of him so I can get on. To tell you the truth, I wait on him hand and foot.'

Her adult son, on the other hand, was 'very good':

'He's very efficient. Very self-sufficient. I never had to make

> his bed. He wouldn't just throw the bedclothes back, either. It was always properly made. And once a week, he'd say, "Give me the clean sheets, Mum," and he'd change his own bed. No, he's very good like that.'

Her health, she described as 'not too good'. She had 'never been robust' and had 'had just about everything'. She had had a hysterectomy in her late twenties after the birth of her third child. The reasons for this had not been made clear to her, and she still wasn't quite sure why she had had it done. She didn't take patent medicines if she felt ill, but would normally rest. If she still felt ill, she would go to the doctor's. She fell into our category of 'high consulters', although she was herself rather critical of patients who often went to the doctor's. Asked how she felt about her children leaving home, she felt that she had coped well, but that her son had been sad to leave, and hadn't really wanted to leave his home and his mum to get married.

This patient, like Mrs. M., who is described below, raises issues linking family and health. These include the pleasures (and otherwise) of the work involved in bringing up children, 'help' in the house from husband and children, and 'work' and 'housework' as differentially conceived and valued activities.

Mrs M. (like other middle-aged patients we spoke to) also alluded to the 'male menopause' and general problems of male health and problems concerning the care of the elderly in a society where 'community care' is seen to be 'A Good Thing' but is frequently simply an overworked daughter, wife or mother providing care for the chronically sick or handicapped in her home.

Mrs M. almost never went to the doctor's. She lived in a council house in the suburbs of a large industrial town, and also left school at 14 and married at 20. She did school cleaning and was a dinner lady 'for mentally handicapped kiddies'. Her husband was a plumber, and her father had done the same thing. After leaving school:

> 'I did church embroidery at a convent. I stayed there till the war started. I married beginning of 1943, and gave up work when I had me daughter. I used to take in work at home, but I had five kiddies, and that kept me quite busy.'

As she pointed out when asked about how much time she spent on housework every day, 'When you've got five kiddies, you're sort of on the trot all the time.' She enjoyed housework, though she would have liked a bit more time and a bit more money to buy things. She got up at 5.45, worked until 9 in the house, went to the school where she worked until 2.30, went back to the school to clean from 4 until 6 and was often still cooking for her sons (now teenagers) at 11 at night. When asked if she got much leisure time, she replied:'I goes out a good bit. I get me old mum's shopping.' Her children helped a bit:

> 'The girls used to when they were at home. The boys are quite capable, but they don't unless you ask them to. If I don't happen to be in when they come in, they'll always get themselves something to eat till I get here, you know. If I'm up me mum's, or down me daughter's babysitting or anything like that.'

She had never been ill ('touch wood') except for one day, and her daughter had looked after the household that day. Her only real anxieties were about her mother. She was failing a bit in health. Should she come and live with them or not? Could she cope on her own? How would she and the children get on if she came to live with the daughter? Her husband, she felt, had taken a rather funny turn as he got older. Could it be the change?

> 'Now, this is an old wives' tale, but all the time I was carrying me kiddies, it was him that had the backaches, it was him that had his eyes – they blacked as if someone had hit him, and it happened more than once, and when he went to work, they said, "What's the matter, Jim, has the wife hit you one?" And they just come up as if he'd had a good hit. And I know that when I was going six months without seeing [a period], it was him that was in a funny mood, and I used to say, "Cor, love us, you've had me children for me and now you're having me change for me."

She missed the children who had left home, but still saw them, and commented that looking after a grandchild was considerably easier than looking after her own children. She would take a tonic if she ever felt under the weather; give her pint of blood; go for 'cancer tests'. She 'wouldn't want a full-time job', since she needed time to look after her mum. Asked whether she thought her children would have the same sort of life as her, she replied with some pride: 'I mean, a couple of my girls have got more now than I've ever had, where the home and all that's concerned, you know. But see, things are different now. You have more now, don't you?' She felt strongly that she was 'very lucky', and put her good health down to three main factors. First, it was being wanted. Her sons would bring her boxes of chocolates, and 'spoil' her (her words): 'It makes my day.' Second, she felt that she had a lot to be thankful for. Her own children, for instance, were all healthy, and so was her grandchild: 'Not like those poor kiddies in the school where I work.' Third, she felt (with some justification) that she was 'too busy' to be affected by minor complaints.

Without being unhappy within the family, both these women contradict the popular view of the family as a haven from the workplace. For most women, *it is* the workplace, in which there are commitments to parents, children, grandchildren and others. The fact that this is usually a labour of love does not mean that these demands do not take their own toll on the health of the carer.

'Taking care of the family means taking care of yourself'

If those who design health education leaflets are correct, it is an awareness of her family commitments which is the most pressing reason why a woman should take care of her own health. Waiting for morning surgery to start one day, I picked up a leaflet in the waiting room. It urged women to attend for cervical screening because: 'TAKING CARE OF THE FAMILY means TAKING CARE OF YOURSELF. If you are ill, you cannot help them. TAKE NO CHANCES. BE SURE!' In its powers of persuasion, the leaflet hit the nail on the head: in so far as women are to take care of themselves it is in order to be able to care for *other* people.

Several women commented on taking action about their own illnesses because of worry about its effect on the rest of the family. One woman, a factory cleaner married to a salesman, had had a hysterectomy three years previously, and had used her savings to go privately because: 'You owe it to your family, don't you, to have these things done quickly if you need them.' Another patient described her nervous breakdown: 'I was right bad with me nerves. I went too late, really, and what made me go was my husband. He were losing weight and that, and he couldn't do anything right as far as I was concerned.' Here, it was concern about the family which took a sick woman to the doctor's. Even if it is the family that makes the patient sick, it is still for the sake of her family that she must get better:

> 'I had a lot of trouble with my daughter and then I had trouble with my husband. I don't say I couldn't face it, or I wouldn't still be here, but it took a lot out of me. 'Cause I went on the drink, but the doctor was very good. . . . But nobody knew . . . the kids never knew. . . . And the more I did it, the more my husband thought I was terrible. I don't drink at all now. But I'd never drunk before, either, not before all this trouble. The doctor wanted me to go and see a psychiatrist or something, but I couldn't face it. I couldn't face that. I think I was ashamed. I knew I was doing wrong and I couldn't stop it. Well, I could stop it . . . but, well, it gives you an awful lot of peace of mind, you know. I drank enough to . . . everything went over the top. It was either that or get out, and I didn't want to get out. The children still needed me.'

In this case, being a good patient meant being a good mother. She became 'sick', went to the doctor for treatment, and this (and the drink) enabled her to stay with her family. But as Stimson and Webb[4] point out, being a 'good' patient may conflict with being a 'good' mother. A 'good' patient doesn't call out the doctor in the night. A 'good' mother may need to. A 'good' mother who might never dream of insisting that she knows her own body better than the doctor may sometimes insist that she knows her child's better, and that something must be done. A patient who may be afraid of the receptionist on her own behalf will be firmer when it comes to her children, perhaps because when she consults for herself, she is a patient; when she consults for her child, she is the primary carer.

Work, housework and 'help'

Once work within the home is accepted as a woman's work, contributions from other household members can only be seen as 'help'. They may do the shopping or cook for meals that they will eat or make their own beds, but they are not seen as helping themselves. They are helping the 'housewife'. However much a woman may protest that she isn't a housewife, or doesn't like the label – 'I'm not married to the house, after all' – there is a real sense in which she is never off duty so long as she is in charge of the household. Other people may do the shopping, but it is her responsibility if there is no sugar in the house. The children may have two parents, but only one of them is to blame if the football shorts haven't been washed. Even for those women who don't have an additional job outside the home, the burden of this unremitting responsibility is unlikely to be good for the health. Even doctors have some time when they are not on call; the same is rarely true for mothers.

A recent letter to a women's magazine from a male reader shows how acceptable it still is for men to be incapable in the home:

> After my wife had given birth to our second daughter we decided that I'd take two weeks holiday to look after four year old Sarah and the house, while my wife concentrated her efforts on the baby and resting. I was eager to show my family how 'together' I could be on the domestic scene, but I was in for a shock. Home was a place I seemed to know nothing about. I didn't know how to operate the washing machine and the igniting mechanism on the oven was beyond me. . . . I also saw for the first time the milkman, doctor, health visitor and grocer.

Not only is it not a matter of shame if a man does not know how to light the oven, it is considered sufficiently amusing to be printed in a women's magazine. At around the same time, there was a letter from a woman reader, under the headline 'Neurotic Women, Noble Men':

> I watched a man on television who was, rightly, very proud

> of his garden – the weed-free vegetable patch and immaculate borders, the smooth green lawns. But what if that man had been a woman, and the garden her home? Would she have been on TV to boast that nowhere in her home was there a speck of dust? That no cushion was out of place, not a dirty mark anywhere? No! She would probably be visiting some psychiatrist (sent, perhaps by her husband!) to find out why she had such a complex about keeping her home neat and tidy. She'd also be on tranquillisers to help her calm down. When it comes to tidiness, is there one law for men and another for women?

For a woman, a tidy house is a matter of duty. To enjoy it as a matter of pride may be seen as neurotic.

Standards don't have to be very high for husband and children to be described as 'good' at helping. One woman explained tolerantly: 'My husband hates cooking. He'd rather starve than cook. But he does do the polishing, and I expect he could do the housework if I was ill or anything, but it would be a bit chaotic.' Another woman, who had married late and at 50 had three children aged 5, 7 and 9, had a husband who would cook. She said, 'He cooks by hisself sometimes and says, "You're lazy." ' One husband had helped in the past, but had given up once his daughters became old enough to give a hand. Just as well, perhaps, that there was someone there to help out, since around the same time, the husband brought a young lad home from work to live with them: 'We took in a lad when he was 15. Frank brought him in from work one day. He didn't have a mum and dad, so he came to live with us.' Mrs L.'s husband had helped out: 'I had a nervous breakdown about three years ago. Me husband looked after me. He were always at the fish and chip shop. Me son cooked me a few meals.'

Some women claim not to want a husband who was too helpful: 'He's not the namby-pamby type, thank God! But if I died tomorrow, he wouldn't go hungry, he could cope.' One woman had had a first husband, a Commanding Officer in the Forces, who had been rather similar to that: 'He didn't lift a finger. Once he sat down at the table, he never got up. I became a batman.' The next husband was a great improvement: 'He'll do whatever you want him to do. He's a damn good man in the house. He'll help with the washing up.' But he does have his drawbacks:

> 'I don't have time to go out in the evening. In fact, my husband, when he comes home at night, having been away all day, he expects me to be here. He brings work home, and I mustn't talk to him. At least, I must sit, be around. . . . I think probably if I'd started much earlier in my marriage insisting on going out in the evenings, I should probably have done it. But he's always expected that I be here all evening, and that's it.'

The demands made by both house and household tend to be high, but there are ways that even the most demanding relationships within the family can be accommodated. Doctor, husband and patient may together define housework and childcare as non-work, or define a woman as being 'too sick to work' long before that definition would be given to a man. Far from being protective, this is a stipulation to the woman that she must conserve her energies to look after the home. One woman told us:

> 'I would have loved to train as a nurse. I would have loved it. But circumstances, you know, haven't allowed it. And perhaps now, when I could, my husband says that my work in the home is far more important, and I would get too involved and I would spend too many hours away. And with the doctor saying I shouldn't work. . . . Well, er, well, it just wouldn't do. Yes, I would have loved to have been a nurse. In fact, I wanted to when I left school, but my mother and father were absolutely against it. But when I decided to join the Red Cross, I thought, "This is a marvellous opportunity, and I'm not going to miss it." And I didn't. That's the only time I've had the courage to put my foot down and say, "Right, I am going to do something I want to do." I went to the hospital for quite a while after that, and then, then something happened with one of my children and I decided they probably needed me at home at lunch-time more than I was needed at the hospital, so I stopped going.'

The idea that the family should come first was well entrenched. One woman who had never given up work outside the home still pointed out:

> 'Although I've always gone out to work, I've never done a job, I can truthfully say, that has ever really affected my family. That they had to come home and do for themselves. I've always managed to work it at least that I've been in, to have a meal ready.'

And while the future General Practitioner is not taught that a mother's going out to work is harmful to children, he is taught that it is the responsibility of the mother (rather than that of the parents) to ensure the care of the child: 'It has never been shown that children are disabled in any important way by having a mother who goes out to work, as long as she makes satisfactory alternative arrangements for them in her brief absences.'[5] It should be said, however, that this passage does appear in a section headed 'parental' rather than 'maternal' deprivation – in itself, a major advance. But the message is that mothers are responsible for ensuring that 'alternative arrangements in her brief absences' are made. Quite what the effect is on children of the absences of a father – often for much longer periods – is not explored. If men are not quite as essential as women to the health of their children, what of their own health? Several of the women we spoke to had observations to make on this.

Looking after men

> 'Men! If they were in a raffle, you wouldn't buy a ticket in case you won one.' (Middle-aged divorced patient.)

One of the major tasks for women is looking after men. Being a mother, both in societies where there is a highly medicalised approach to childbirth and in societies where there is not, makes demands on a woman's health. Being a wife also takes its toll, and certainly makes demands on a woman's time. Some of the middle-aged women we spoke to had some interesting observations to make about men, some of which we have already seen in the context of ageing, and about 'explanations' of illness in relation to men and women. Some harsh judgments were made on men by some of the women we spoke to – often, as far as one could tell, with good reason. There were several women who had fallen foul of the cruelly different way that ageing is perceived among men and among women, and who had, it seemed, been 'traded in' for a younger model.[6] One deserted wife said: 'After his mother died, I though he was getting ill, but no, he was turning wicked.' Another kept her end up: 'They go through a sort of menopause themselves. They tend to tart themselves up a bit. But God, you wouldn't have been attracted to them when they were 20, let alone 40 or 50.'

A woman who devotes her life to looking after her children and looking after her husband, one who has perhaps given up or not taken a job at her husband's insistence, may well find herself abandoned – sometimes because the husband claims to feel himself 'trapped', or because he wants a more 'independent' woman. She experiences redundancy in a particularly poignant manner. Where do you go for help, advice, for sympathy if this sort of thing happens to you? All the doctors we spoke to mentioned the 'deserted wife' or the wife with the unfaithful husband, as a problem. Some of the women could openly discuss marital difficulties with the doctor. Others, perhaps feeling that this was not an appropriate entrée to the doctor's surgery, would become ill and need attention. These sorts of situations, according to one doctor, did not happen very often, but when they did, they were very dramatic:

> 'You remember them. . . . There are floods of tears, and, you know, they're tearing their handkerchief to ribbons, and their husband's just gone off with the secretary or some dollybird or something. But it doesn't happen every week, every month. It happens perhaps twice a year, and perhaps not that. But you remember, partly because it's so dramatic, and partly because it tends to start off a long series of visits, you know.'

There is little that even the caring doctor can do for the woman in this situation. He or she is hardly likely to be able to bring the erring husband back. Any 'treatment' is likely to define the woman (rather than her wandering husband) as the problem, and yet it is still apparently rare for doctors in this situation to step outside the medical model.

When contemplating marriage, young women should, perhaps, be advised to think of the risk to their health.

Madness is hereditary: you catch it from your children

As we have seen, the 'empty nest syndrome' can be used as an explanation for ill-health in middle age, but women's feelings about their children leaving home vary widely. One woman was painfully aware of the effect that her attachment to children had had on the rest of her life:

> 'I still want to be amongst children. I'm not – to be honest – I'm not happy amongst grown-ups. I get tongue-tied. . . . If there's a party, I end up in the kitchen making sandwiches . . . I don't mind. I'd like to come in the front, but I can't, it's no good. I'd like to work with children, but I don't think you could without qualifications. I don't think I'd go for company amongst grown-ups. I've never felt as if I'm a prisoner, but I'm beginning to. I begin to feel that I'm fastened in. . . . My family's growing away, and I'm beginning just to feel it. Oh, I don't resent them going away or anything, but I'm beginning to feel I should have had more than just my family. I begin to realise it now – that I should have had outside interests'.

Another woman had similar feelings, but for different reasons: 'When they were little, like, it was better. Now, they expect to burden their mother with all their troubles. They don't realise you've got troubles of your own'. Another said: 'It's nice to have a bit of peace.'

A West Indian woman who was often at the doctor's felt that her children should take some blame for her poor health. When they were young, she had worked as a night nurse. She was a respectable, God-fearing woman. Her children's radicalism and dissatisfaction were hard for her to take:

'I'd like to go back to work. I'm really desperate to work, but I'm not really right in my body because of the worry about the kids. . . . When they were small, it was much better. Now they tangle your heart. Your heart's in sorrows all the time. . . . They live their own life [though they were living with her]. I want them to get a profession, but they don't want to listen, they don't want to know.'

The children's father was in the West Indies, but, she said, 'Even if he was here, I'd want a job, my own money. I like my independence. But my girls aren't like that. They want to be looked after by the boys.'

Not all mothers, however, encouraged this attutide. Mrs B., a woman who had not had a particularly happy marriage, told us:

'My daughter's courting. She's been going out with this lad for ten weeks now. But she said to me the other day, "Mum, I don't want to get married. I don't fancy cooking and cleaning every day. I'd rather be as I am." Mind you, she's not very mature for her age. I expect she'll change.'

It is not only ill-health or patterns of visiting the doctor which are reproduced within families. Patterns of behaviour can also be reproduced. Has the daughter who was 'not very mature for her age' changed? Is she now cooking and cleaning, too? If some women, like this one, are threatened by daughters who want a different kind of life (or perhaps can realistically see just how difficult it is to break the mould), others see a more fulfilling life for their daughters. Mrs P. told us:

'My daughter does her own decorating. I had the frustration of never being able to do that, because my husband said, "That's my job. You've got your jobs, and I've got my jobs. . . ." My daughter will have a better life than me, although mine hasn't been really unhappy. Frustrating, perhaps, but not unhappy.'

Most of the women we spoke to had children who were growing up. As one of them said: 'The books that tell you how to look after children stop when they get to school age. That's the easy bit. The responsibility still goes on. As long as you're alive, you still worry.'

Care of the elderly

The women we spoke to were involved not only in the health care of their husbands and children, but frequently, too, in the care of their parents, parents-in-law, or elderly neighbours. Some were shocked by the force with which they were hit by the death of their mothers. Mrs W. remembered: 'My mother died eight years ago. We were real pals, my mum and me, and we had just moved. I had a sort of nervous breakdown then.'

Another woman felt that her own ill-health had been brought about by her mother's death:

> 'My mother died last January, and I became awfully sad after that and this winter, I've caught all sorts of things which usually I never do. Usually, I'm in very good health. . . . I never thought it would affect me so badly. She had lived with us for years, and was very sprightly for 88. She never saw the doctor – she had a horror of doctors. She did have bronchitis, which gave her a bit of trouble with her breathing, and the doctor did warn me that it would put an extra strain on her heart. I'd always thought I would accept it when she did go, and in a way, it wasn't so bad for the first few weeks. It was afterwards, really. I stopped going to meet my friends for lunch. People would say, "Oh, she had a good life, and it was the best way to go," which was true, I suppose, but I found it difficult to accept. And no one ever talks about it except to say that. I could never talk to my family about it. My husband doesn't believe in talking, he thinks that when things happen, you should forget them, not drag them out. I often wonder if I'm funny, being so sad about it. After all, it's a long time, isn't it, last January?'

Coming at the same time, often, as the children leaving home, the death of a parent seemed particularly hard to take. Mrs D. made the link between the two events:

> 'I missed them [the children], but they were happy, I did go through a period when I felt right sorry for meself, and when the last got married, I thought, "Now, what are you

going to do with the rest of your life?" And Frank's dad died round about the same time, and I'd thought a right lot about his dad, and looked after him and that.'

One of the few 'stories' which verged on being a complaint about a doctor arose in the context of looking after an elderly parent. Mrs F. had looked after her elderly mother:

'She wasn't totally bedridden, but I had been tied for eleven years, you see. Really tied. She'd had heart trouble, and the doctor realised I was on the verge of breaking down, I think, and she was taken into hospital for sort of three weeks so we could go on holiday, which was the first break, really, I'd had, and, er, she actually was kept in hospital a little bit longer and she died there. . . . I suppose I did go through a pretty bad patch . . . but I'm pretty resilient really. We were very close, but it was a mercy she died, if you know what I mean. . . . It was rather a distressing business, really, because the doctor, he was very good, he got her into hospital to give her this break and um, we were, well, my husband and I were absolutely on the edge. We'd never asked for any help before, she'd never been away or anything. . . . We never asked for anything. . . . She'd got Parkinson's disease, which we hadn't known. We asked if she could stay and I don't think we had very good treatment, really, because we had to go and see the registrar. . . . He was very kind, but he upset my husband terribly because he said – he was a very nice man, I've nothing against him at all – but he turned to my husband and said, "Well, why didn't you put her in a home years ago?" Well, my husband, he nearly collapsed in tears. . . .

I couldn't get used to going out and not having to tear back. Oh, it took me a long time to get used to that. But I was free . . . and for once able to put myself first instead of always last. . . . My husband . . . he was so . . . we've got to do what's right, type of thing, It's our job, I mean, the nurse used to say, anyone would think it's his mother. I had to look after her. It was right and proper. And I'd never queried it, really. He [the GP] was *very* understanding. He saw us actually after his surgery, and he's often late. And we were there a very long time. And he was very, very helpful. . . . I didn't lean on my husband. Well, I have to lean on myself. I was the king pin, really. I was the strongest one there. . . . I think it's perhaps wrong to go to the doctor's. They're too busy. I think it's a great pity that you can't, but I don't feel that you should in today's sort of circumstances. . . . I had to go to him because I couldn't sleep, but, my goodness me, it took me a long time to go. I had to be very desperate to go. There had to be a real reason.'

This patient raises several questions in relation to illness and the family. Had the patient been 'too strong' in battling on until she was on the verge of a nervous breakdown, or not strong enough? Had she done the right thing by her mother? With these questions in her mind, and the undoubted suspicion that something was wrong somewhere, she was still unwilling really to criticise the medical profession. The hospital doctor, in spite of everything, was 'a very nice man, I've nothing against him at all.' He may have almost reduced her husband to tears, but he did, after all, take the mother in. The GP was pretty good, too. He had given time after surgery to talk. But this woman had given eleven years of her life to the full-time care of an elderly and chronically ill parent and had only sought help when she was on the verge of a breakdown. The contradictions concerning her own time, the nature and value of her work and the effects of this work on her own health do not seem to have been explored by patient, doctor or husband. To what extent do doctors see the family or the household as a workplace? And, in particular, a place where health work takes place? There is, after all, a good deal more caring for the sick and maintaining the healthy in the home than in the hospital or health centre.

How do doctors see families and the place of women within them? How do they act in ways which sustain their preconceptions, and how do women themselves view and respond to their positions as wives, mothers and workers, their own varied experiences, and the conduct of doctors? Both women and doctors were likely to hold the view that illness interfered with the caring capacity of the housewife; there was far less sense that illness might be *caused* by it. But there could therefore be a conflict between the notion of a good patient, who would not consult on her own behalf because she did not want to 'bother' the doctor, and the good housewife, who would, because she did not want to fail in her duties to her dependants. One should not look for absolute consistency, either in the views of women as a whole, or in those of particular groups of women. Indeed, it is the presence of incompatible, or potentially incompatible, views and experiences which provides the possibility for change. But only the possibility. Lack of consistency on the part of doctors is likely to result only in contradictory prescriptions for their patients.

A doctor may well realise that Valium is not what the deserted wife needs, but what else can he or she prescribe within the current structures? Perhaps his or her own time, to listen, to sympathise, to counsel for the future. But given the organisation of surgery time, the patient is likely to get at best a confusing mixture – as much time as the doctor can spare, and because he or she realises that it isn't enough, a prescription, too. While ambivalence in doctors concerning their women patients can lead to confusion, a similar ambivalence in patients is likely to lead to anxiety, tension and illness. Being a good mother, a good wife, a good worker and a good doctor is a tall order.

It remains women who care and nurture. *They* are responsible for health within the family – for childcare, general health, ill-health and the care of the elderly. These heavy responsibilities may well take their toll on a woman's own health. Given a body of working beliefs (held by patients as well as by doctors) which constantly 'create' women as functional to someone else (get better so you can look after your family), women may be deprived even of the dignity to be ill in their own right.

Chapter 6

Making changes

Making changes poses contradictions. Within limits, the patients are happy – 'He's a lovely man.' Similarly, the doctors (if we ignore their higher-than-average rates of alcoholism, depression and suicide) are not totally miserable with the way that things are at present. Still, there is also a 'but . . .', sometimes spoken and sometimes unspoken, in both doctors' and women's accounts of the consultation: 'He's a lovely man, but . . .'; 'I do my best for my patients, but. . . .' If we believe that there is something wrong with the present structure of doctor–patient relationships, what sort of changes could be made?

The most radical of radical views normally suggests that small changes are 'liberal'; that they may even be counter-productive in that they allow the current system to accommodate dissatisfactions without any 'real' change; that until there is complete change, we might as well have no change. This, however, tends to be the view of the generals directing movements of social change. For them, the fact that the infantry are having a bad time in the here and now is just one of those things we have to put up with in the interests of revolutionary transformation.

Another view is that it's worth making what changes we can, when we can. That if we wait for 'the moment', we might have a long wait. And women patients might not want to be all that patient. We should also bear in mind that small changes are taking place in any system all the time. And there's a good chance that if these changes aren't taking place in the direction we might choose, they're taking place in someone else's; serving someone else's interests.

One example of change that doesn't necessarily suit the patients is the change in surgery hours in some practices, with less and less (and sometimes no) time allocated to evening surgery. Another example is the increasing use of deputising services, with deputising doctors covering vast areas and attending patients whose history they do not know. On the more positive side, some doctors have made changes greatly to the benefit of patients. One South Coast doctor, for instance, runs late-evening surgeries after her children are settled for the night – a move which also suits many of her patients. Other practices have allocated a room on the premises as a creche, so that if there are long waits, they are less uncomfortable, both for the very young and for the waiting patients whose tolerance of healthy boisterous toddlers may be reduced by their own ill-health. Some doctors make it clear to parents of young children who may dither about whether or not to 'bother' a doctor that they are always willing to chat on the phone to help a parent come to a decision about whether to call out a doctor, come to the surgery or simply give a junior aspirin. (Naturally, this telephone service is only really useful if it is an addition to, rather than a substitute for, face-to-face dealings with patients.) Some practices have a library where patients may borrow books about pregnancy, childbirth, self-help or picture books for children about to go into hospital.

These are by no means revolutionary changes. For the patient patients, though, one hundred small changes in the here and now are better than the faint glimmer of hope of complete change at some time in the dim and distant future. Indeed, the small changes may well be preferable. During a discussion with a sensitive and caring General Practitioner of some of the very conservative opinions of the patients in this book, he pointed out that the women had good reason to be suspicious of change. The present system could be coped with; it was understood. It was the patients, not the ideologists who would be the first to be affected by changes. And if changes went wrong, or were difficult to cope with, it was they who suffered.

But if practical changes are both possible and desirable, what should be their general direction? For to make significant changes now is not simply to alter in a random or haphazard manner. The changes outlined above, for instance, are by no means random: surgery hours are normally changed in order to improve the working conditions of those running, not those attending, the surgeries; deputising services similarly benefit the doctor more than the patient. These changes reflect the fact that doctors as a group are more organised than patients. Where patients do get together and organise for change, doctors may be antagonistic; but things do begin to change . . . slowly. Would there have been such changes in maternity services in the last few years without pressure groups such as Aims and the National Childbirth Trust? Almost certainly not, whatever the efforts of good individuals within the system.

A major impetus for change in issues concerning women's health has been the women's health movement, which in this country developed mainly around the campaign for free abortion. It has now broadened its scope – making information on women's health more widely available, campaigning on the availability and safety of different methods of contraception, providing feminist approaches to therapy, fertility and other areas affecting the health of women.

The clear message of the women's health movement has been that health must be delivered back into the hands of those most directly affected by health. And these are not the doctors, but ourselves. This impetus does, of course, have the potential, as activists in the women's movement are well aware, of being interpreted in the most conservative of ways. To say that health must be in our own hands is a very different matter from saying that people are to blame for their own ill-health, and if only they ate more yoghurt and did more yoga all would be well. The Health Education Council's expensive Look After Yourself campaign came dangerously close to suggesting that people become ill because they're careless. A further danger contained in taking responsibility for one's own health is that it carries the potential problem that those who can 'purchase' a best buy can get it. The rest can look after themselves with cocoa and elastoplast.

This should not be taken to imply that you get a better standard of surgery or medicine if you pay for it – the reverse may be the case. But in areas like continuity of care, one way of ensuring you always see the same doctor for ante-natal care (for instance) is, unfortunately, to pay for it. And the 'best buy' may not simply be a financial transaction, in any case. In many cases, it is knowledge and not the purse which is power.

To suggest, then, that we take more responsibility for our own health is not to suggest that we take it over ourselves – setting up neighbourhood heart surgery clinics or do-it-yourself kidney transplants. The heroic intervention of surgery, after all, is relevant to only a minute proportion of our health needs. Perhaps the greatest step in this direction is for women to redefine themselves as basically healthy.

This is an enormous task, but great steps forward have already been made. Women are more and more reluctant to see themselves as patients when they are pregnant or giving birth. They do not, on the whole, define themselves as 'sick' when they are menstruating. Far from it being fashionable to be a weak, swooning creature, looking and being healthy is a priority, if features in women's magazines are anything to go by. Of course, there are some counter-currents. The 'discovery' of pre-menstrual tension is not good news for most women, and may well encourage women (and their doctors) to adopt biological explanations for socially induced misery, anxiety or dissatisfaction. Snapping at your husband? At your wits' end with the children? It could all be PMT. Women should not allow themselves to be defined as sick simply because the way they live and the way they are treated would be enough to make anyone sick. As Ann Oakley has recently pointed out: 'Women's energies in our kind of society appear to be devoted to "doing good and feeling bad".'[1]

The problem is not that women cannot cope, but that they are put in situations which are intolerable, and which should, and can, be changed. To define things in this way makes it clear that the woman is an actor within a bad set of arrangements, rather than a sufferer of them. At the same time, redefinition both increases her power of self-control and makes realistic the possibility of a 'cure'. Ann Oakley[2] argues that the medicalisation of depression has been one of the greatest disasters women have experienced this century. This defines women as ill, rather than defining their situation as intolerable. We need to make redefinitions a part of our strategy for change.

For women to redefine themselves as basically healthy is, however, to take a risk, and one which women patients are clearly well aware of. As things are, their only chance of getting a break is to be 'sick' – only then do they get some of the nurturing that they constantly give: to be totally healthy is to be totally active and never to have a break. Redefining oneself as healthy only makes sense if other parts of one's life and responsibilities are redefined, too.

In many senses, this has been what the women's movement, and particularly consciousness-raising sessions, has been about. Women who feel unhappy or dissatisfied with a 'nice home, doting husband, lovely kids' are somewhat less likely now to think that they, and not the sorts of lives they lead, are to blame for their feelings. The kinds of changes which might be made in the here and now are discussed below – first, as they might come from the doctors' side, and then from the patients'.

The doctors' side

Seven years ago, an article by 'Dr Wimpole' appeared in a popular women's magazine. The subject was cystitis:[3]

> 'I've got cystitis again,' or 'These antibiotics have given me thrush', are phrases I hear every day. And these diagnoses are often very wrong. What the girl [sic] should say is, 'My urine hurts and I keep wanting to go all the time,' or 'I've got an itchy discharge. Do you think it might be caused by the Tetracycline you gave me for that throat infection last week?'

What is interesting about this is not so much the patronising attitude, the characterisation of the patient as a 'girl', the reluctance to hear the patient using 'grown-up' terms like cystitis ('I keep wanting to go to go all the time,' keeps her firmly in her place), but rather the fact that only a few years later, such an article would not be printed. 'Dr Wimpole' has been superannuated and replaced by a doctor who is more in keeping with the times, who does not refer to the readers of *Woman's Own* as 'girls'. His articles are more informative, more discursive, less patronising. It would be unrealistic to ask – to politely suggest, perhaps – to a powerful group that they give up some of their power. Why should they? But things are moving a little. People will move when pushed, as the changes in the maternity services show. What sort of changes might one see from doctors?

The training of doctors

> Perhaps the most important attribute of a competent doctor is that he [sic] knows what he can do and what he cannot do. . . . The man who considers he is competent over the whole field, whatever his previous experience and however many diplomas he has obtained, is a public nuisance.[4]

The problem with general practice is that doctors do have to be generalists, do have to have a wide sphere of competence, and are expected to exercise their intellects over a wide sphere – only a part of which they have been trained for.

To suggest a change in the types of students entering medical school is perhaps the most liberal of liberal reforms. To believe that there would be any great change by having more women students, more mature students, more students from a working-class background, more students who began their careers as nurses or laboratory technicians or physiotherapists, would be to underestimate the socialising power of medical schools. Students are not merely taught medicine at medical schools – they are taught what it means to be a doctor: how doctors dress; how they address patients and nurses; and what 'counts' as important information.

None the less, though a change in the composition of medical students would not bring about revolution, it might bring some changes. Mature students are more likely to challenge their teachers, since they have their own experiences to offer. More working-class students would present another sort of challenge. As for women, it has been suggested that it might be an easier task to teach those who care to become doctors, than to teach doctors to care. Although the current entry to medical schools in Britain is now around 50 per cent women, quotas were only abolished in the 1960s, and there is still an uneasy acceptance of women in the profession as a whole. Fifty per cent of students are women, but what of registrars and consultants? In 1977,[5] fewer than 10 per cent of consultants were women, about 19 per cent of senior registrars, and about 18 per cent of registrars. A recent editorial in the *British Medical Journal* refers to women's careers as doctors:[6]

> Any woman doctor who decides to make a career in a prestigious speciality such as neurology or cardiothoracic surgery will find that she is competing with men who give 100% of their effort to their work: she cannot expect to succeed if she tries to combine her specialist training with bringing up a family herself. It would be quite wrong for any modification to be made to the existing system to encourage part-time training in such demanding branches of medicine, for standards would inevitably fall.

As one geriatrician pertinently asked in a subsequent letter to the journal, why is it that heart surgery is considered more 'demanding' than care of the elderly?[7] The article concludes: 'What is wanted in the NHS is practical provision for the needs of women who wish to combine medicine with marriage without damage to the standards of either.'[8] Men, apparently are able to marry without damage to either patients or career. Are they perhaps expected to remain childless? Or do their children not suffer from paternal deprivation? In advocating more places for women medical students, one would not be advocating a drop in standards. Far from it. Women normally do better in their examinations. Nor are they significantly more likely to leave the profession than their male colleagues. Beulah Bewley and Thomas Bewley, writing in the *Lancet* in 1975 point out that:[9]

> Women doctors who temporarily and partially drop out of full-time practice have been studied frequently, but men (who are equally expensive to train) have not, despite their disappearing from National Health Service practice through emigration, death, alcoholism, suicide or removal from the Medical Register. In a working lifetime of forty years, a women doctor with an average family is likely to

> do seven-eighths of the work of a doctor who has not had to carry the primary responsibility of bearing and rearing children.

The following advert, however, placed by a group practice in a national newspaper, does suggest that things can change, if only very slowly.[10]

> FEMINIST DOCTOR
>
> Wanted from 1st January 1982 as part time assistant to join expanding NHS GP practice. Skill in Women's Health, Child Development and Obstetrics valued.
>
> We are a radical collective committed to holistic health care. . . .

Would such an advertisement have appeared without the presence of a women's health movement? Almost certainly not. One can expect that under certain circumstances, doctors will respond to, or participate in, movements for social change. Changes of this sort are not self-generating.

Health education

When the National Health Service was first set up, it was expected that costs would initially be very high but would eventually fall as the national back-log of ill-health was cleared and the nation as a whole became fitter. The reverse has happened – demand has gone up. Attempts at health education have been ragged. Educating patients is not normally seen as part of the GP's work,[11] and apart from a few Health Education Council posters in the waiting room, patients may often complete their transaction in the surgery with little learning on either side.

Patients cannot be expected to take responsibility for their health if they have only the vaguest idea what is going on in their bodies, what medications they are taking and why, what operation they have had and what the effects are. We found many beliefs and fears about illness based upon misconceptions, even though the women we spoke to were, as it happens, patients in practices where the doctors were, to a greater or lesser extent, patient-centred, and did talk to their patients. But this clearly wasn't enough.

All the women were quite intelligent enough to understand their own health more fully, if only the doctors and patients could communicate better. One woman we interviewed had had a hysterectomy:

> 'I had all my womb taken away, and they took away all the . . . now . . . what did they take away? Well, they took everything away, I think. And then they injected me with . . . a hormone, is it? And that started me on the change of life.'

Another woman in hospital with depression had been given ECT:

> 'Well, she brought me this form to sign and I said, "What's this for, I'm not having no operation." And she said, "No, you're not. It's for ECT." "Well," I said, "what's that?" And she said, "You'll find out." Well, I was given ECT[12] and it was quite nice. Being in that hospital, it was the nicest time I'd had for a long time. You should try it.'

We frequently came across the idea that heavy periods were 'good', since they got rid of all the 'bad' blood. A woman who had had problems with this over several years said: 'I'd rather suffer a bit with the menopause, because then you know that you've got rid of all that. Whereas if you just stop in later life, you think, "Where did all that go?" Even among the most educated patients, there were misconceptions about what antibiotics can usefully be prescribed for, what it means to have a virus, what happens to your periods after a hysterectomy, whether you still ovulated, and so on. If they were being given explanations, these were not being understood. One doctor laughingly told us about his explanations to patients:

> 'I think in a practice with people who are, er, more sophisticated – you know, teachers and things – they do require a lot of explanations for what you are doing, you know. Or they get it, even if they don't want it, you know, you tend to say, "I must explain to him. . . ." And then there are other families – I mean, if you explain one thing

to them, it's no good going on and on because they just don't take it in. This makes different demands.'

While it is 'common sense' to believe that some groups of patients may be more receptive than others to explanations of ill-health, drugs and treatment, the enormous popularity right across the social spectrum of programmes on health – even on such subjects as triple-bypass surgery – indicates that there are very few patients who would not understand at least the fundamentals of their ill-health. The best time to teach people about their health may not be when they are at their most sick, though sometimes this may be the only course.

Two health courses have recently been set up by a women's health group in Keighley, West Yorkshire. The women who come along are from all walks of life. One course is for those with good or native English; another is run for Asian women with little or no English, for whom the course is run with an interpreter. Twenty two-hour sessions are given on topics ranging from ante-natal care to weight problems, stress and cancer. All sessions are run by a feminist doctor, though other groups running similar courses successfully use lay people with expertise in a particular area. The women also learn to use a stethoscope and sphygmomanometer – not because they are going to become barefoot doctors, but in order to help demystify standard surgery equipment. There are sessions in counselling, assertiveness training, and the sorts of local knowledge that you might need to help make an informed choice about where to go or what to do about a health problem. The course has a good creche, the atmosphere is relaxed. A good deal of time is spent talking about personal experiences of ill-health, relating these to doctors' explanations, and sometimes using them to challenge these explanations. The women who come to these courses are receiving a kind of training; one which will enable them to be a resource themselves for friends and neighbours. Learning is more likely to take place in this sort of atmosphere than when you're in the surgery, not feeling too good, perhaps a bit anxious about the long queue outside, with your child whimpering to go home. And without a better knowledge of their own bodies and their health, how can women take charge?

Medical records and health diaries

> 'I can't quite remember when my periods stopped. Was it last. . . . No. I don't remember. But the doctor will tell you. He's got it written down. It's on my card.'

Knowledge is power. Our medical records are guarded with some secrecy, and the horror expressed, particularly in hospitals, when patients look at their own records, belies the fact that these records are about our bodies and our lives. One could foresee several changes for the better if patients were given their own records by the receptionist to take in to the doctor, and therefore were able, if they wished, to read them. First, the more extreme objectifications of the patient would almost certainly be avoided by GP and consultant alike. It is likely too (though by no means certain), that access by a patient to her own records would encourage doctors to separate the medical from the social – at least in what they write down. The knowledge that there could be some comeback from the patient could well lead the doctor to reflect a little more carefully before writing on the card judgments or comments which will follow the patient round for the rest of her life, however many times she may change her doctor. The power of labelling a patient is considerable. Once a 'neurotic' a 'trouble-maker' a 'difficult patient' a 'hysteric', it is difficult to lose those labels.

But should it always be the doctor who is custodian of the record, or of the whole record, in any case? A Danish GP, Carsten Jespersen, is currently experimenting with health diaries kept by patients themselves. As he points out, if it is a patient who keeps the doctor waiting momentarily while she looks something up in her health diary, this can be a substantial transference of power. (Jespersen does, however, point out that the system can be (ab)used by doctors to increase their knowledge of, and control over, a patient's behaviour, checking the diary to make sure that she has carried out 'doctor's orders').[13] But keeping a health diary, while having some disadvantages (not all patients may have or want to spend time in this way), may make particular sense to someone with a chronic illness, or who has been through a traumatic life event. It can give the patient the opportunity to reflect on her illness, to see that she is perhaps feeling better than this time last week, last year, or five years ago. That this can also be part of a valuable learning process for both doctor and patient is discussed in more detail below.

Learning from the patient

In Britain, there is now a compulsory training scheme for General Practitioners which normally takes three years. This period includes twelve (or sometimes eighteen) months as a trainee in general practice, under the tutelage of a GP. It is clear, however, that it is the General Practitioner who is the trainer, not the patients – though patients have a great deal of knowledge which doctors could usefully share and learn from. How many doctors know what it is like to be a young diabetic or to have multiple sclerosis, to be defined as infertile, or to suffer post-natal depression? Some doctors, of course, will know from their own experience, but this will be rare. Medical textbooks and clinical practice may detail the symptoms, diagnoses, prognoses and treatment of disease, but they rarely explain what it is like to *have* that disease, how patients *feel* about their treatment, their diagnosis and prognosis.

One way in which doctor–patient communication could be improved would be for the doctor to put her or himself frankly in the position of learner. To take one example used earlier: when the ante-natal patient asked the male doctor what it felt like when the baby first moved, instead of giving her an authoritative reply, or even saying, 'Well, I'm a man, I can't really tell you,' he might have said, 'Well, you would be doing me a favour if you wrote down what it feels like to you when you think the baby moves.' Not only might he learn something, since different women have very different experiences of what it feels like when they first feel the baby move, but he would also be validating her as the expert on her own pregnancy.

Doctors could learn from other accounts given by patients. Patients suffering from particular chronic complaints might write down what it feels like to be them. Patients who have suffered a traumatic event (a stillbirth, an accident, a mastectomy) might be encouraged to write their experiences – not only to provide more information about the illness, but to show the ways in which what appear to be very minor interventions by medical personnel might make all the difference between a good and a bad experience. Writing something down can also be therapeutic for the patient. In some recent work concerning miscarriage, for instance,[14] many women ended their accounts by saying how much better they felt after they had written something down. They also felt that their experience was more bearable if there was any chance that it might help someone else to know about it. The fact that many of them were not used to writing made no difference to the eloquence with which they expressed themselves.

For doctors to admit that they have something to learn from their patients' accounts would be a significant change. And they would learn not only about the illness, the complaint, the problem, but also a good deal about the patient. And if the patient were confident enough to be frank about what the doctor had said or done, he might learn something about himself and his own practice.

Well Women Clinics

There is clearly more scope for people to learn about their health when they are well than when they are sick. In some areas, Well Women Clinics have been set up under the National Health Service with the following aims:[15]

> to provide an informal atmosphere in which women feel free to talk about any problems they have;
> to provide more time than is available in the general surgery;
> to attract women who do not normally come to the surgery and who would otherwise feel inhibited about coming to the doctor;
> to screen women for breast and cervical cancer;
> to teach self-examination and self-help for simple problems;
> to train other health workers in the ideas and techniques of Well Women check ups;
> to initiate discussion groups about health topics;
> to increase women's knowledge about health and about the health service.

While the aims may vary a little from one clinic to another (some, for instance, feel that there is insufficient evidence to support breast screening in pre-menopausal women), the general aim remains the same: an emphasis on informality and plenty of time per patient. The clinics are very popular with women – they travel up to forty miles to the open-access clinics in Islington. Although Well Women Clinics only partially meet the problem of women being too intimidated to go to their GP with some problems, it is better that this need be partly met than not met at all. A Liverpool GP who helps to run a Well Women Clinic in her practice describes a woman who felt able to go to the Well Women Clinic but not to the GP's surgery:[16]

> 'One woman mentioned sheepishly that she had been trying desperately to get pregnant for eighteen months, but hadn't dared mention it before, as she was 35 and had two children. She thought we would think she ought to be "past that sort of thing". But she was really keen to have another child. She is now undergoing investigations for secondary infertility.'

It has often been pointed out that the National Health Service is, in effect, a national sickness service, since the majority of services it provides do not concern health but sickness. The Well Women Clinic, like the Well Baby Clinic and Well Child Clinic run in some practices, emphasises that doctors are not just concerned with illness, but with health. And so are patients, for it is only when women become active subjects in the promotion of their own health – rather than passive objects of the merely professional treatment of illness – that any great changes will be made.

Patients' groups

One area where changes have been made, and patients have given one another enormous support, has been in the setting up of patients' groups. There are now patient-support groups for almost every illness; groups for parents whose children are seriously ill; groups for women who are having problems in conceiving or maintaining a pregnancy; groups dealing with both mental and physical ills. In many cases, these groups are patient-initiated. And not only do they provide emotional support, but they may also make significant contributions to discussions concerning the management and treatment of problems. In some cases, however, they are, or could be doctor-initiated.

In Chapter 3, a woman doctor described two patients, each anxious about her son's forthcoming marriage. Could they have supported one another? We saw many women, sometimes within a few hundred yards of one another, who had been deeply shocked by the force with which their mothers' deaths had hit them. Some found it extremely reassuring to be told of other women we had spoken to who felt the same way. Perhaps they, too, had they known each other, could have given support.

Some practices have initiated patients' groups to allow patients a voice in the organisation of the practice. Are surgery hours more convenient for the doctors or for the patients? Would it be possible to have a woman doctor in on a sessional basis to do the ante-natal clinics? Other practices run evenings for particular groups of patients identified by means of the age/sex register. Women who might be interested in a discussion of the menopause, for instance, can be relatively easily identified, and patients we spoke to who had been to such a discussion had found it useful – though the doctors involved felt that the patients tended to be very reticent and to let the doctors run the show.

Groups could be more widely used, as indeed they are in some practices. Groups for patients who have suffered from heart attacks, who have diabetes, who have multiple sclerosis, or even simply for patients who are in the same age group and who might be experiencing the same non-medical life events – such groups could be set up by doctors trained in groupwork. For doctors to lead such groups is not to ignore the potential problems of medical definition and control, but it is the doctor who initially holds all the cards. She or he knows which patients fall into which groups, and any doctor willing to make the effort to set up such a group might well be the sort of person to inspire trust in patients. Patients in such a group could not only help one another by discussing common problems – perhaps diet, perhaps fear – but could also educate the doctor on the real problems of their condition. If the groups are eventually led by patients, so much the better. Meantime, the skills learnt by doctors in leading groups may be helpful in many contexts – in medical politics, or in teaching trainee GPs within the practice.

The patients' side

But what of the patients? To paraphrase Barbara Ehrenreich and Deirdre English, women patients do not unite and fight. Feeling sick, being ill, going to the doctor's – these are essentially solitary activities. For the powerless, seizing power is almost as difficult as persuading the powerful to cede it. We *want* our doctors to be right; we *want* to like her or him; we *want* to believe that we are being treated as adults. It is much easier to rely on the authority of an expert, than to talk to a wide range of people, including one's 'old wife' friends. To treat the doctor as one expert amongst many involves the frightening task of taking on power oneself.

There are various pieces of advice which are often given in relation to a visit to someone powerful – a lawyer, the police, a doctor. Take a friend to even things up a bit; be quietly and politely insistent; make a list to refer to; ask the doctor (lawyer, policeman) questions; write things down if they're important or you think you might forget them. But all this is often easier said than done – one raised eyebrow when you go into the consulting room with a friend may be enough to banish all your good resolutions. Anxious glances from the GP at your long list may cause you to abandon it. It is difficult to be insistent about a particular problem if the doctor is being reassuring and you want to be told that everything is all right. What other resources does the patient have in this situation? One possibility is to remember that the doctor is a person who has a life outside his or her work as a doctor, and to use this fact in the consultation. He or she can be reminded from time to time of her or his role as a 'normal' human being by being asked, 'What would you do if this were you/your wife/your husband/your mother/your child?' This may not affect the sort of advice you are given, but for a moment at least it allows you as a patient to step out of the patient role and the doctor to step out of the role of doctor – for the patient and the doctor to relate to one another as equals, with similar cares, worries and concerns outside the consulting room.

Learning about health

One of the things which makes women patients – perhaps all patients – so powerless when they go to the doctor's is the fact that the doctor is assumed to hold all the knowledge about the patient's body, what symptoms can mean, what treatment would be appropriate. The publication of the women's health book *Our Bodies Ourselves*[17] has had an enormous impact – both on the women who have read it and, through a 'domino' effect, on many other women. Health journalists, having read the book, sense the climate of the times. Women's magazine articles are no longer of the 'Dr Wimpole' type. Many are extremely informative, giving facts and advice about previously taboo subjects such as hysterectomy and mastectomy, and about less serious procedures such as treatments for allergies and the necessity of rubella vaccinations for teenage girls. One rather timid patient proudly described her experience after having read an article on Hormone-Replacement Therapy.

> Years ago, there was an article in the evening paper on the women's page about it, and it said they'd found this new drug that was really good. I wrote it down, and I went to the doctor the next day. Well, I'd been terrible with hot flushes and that, I couldn't stand it, and I thought, well, I'll try this. You never know. And I went there and he said, 'You're quick off the mark aren't you? They've hardly made this drug yet.' and I'd written down what it was called, and I told him what it was, and he said, 'Well, you've spelt it wrong' but he did give it to me. And then I took it to the chemist. Well, that was embarrassing too. Because right in front of everyone, he said, 'You must be the first person in Newtown to be getting this. We haven't even got it in stock yet' – this was Boots – 'but we'll have it in by the end of the week' he said, and they did.

Though the use of HRT may be controversial, there's no doubt that new writing on the subject of health can empower the woman patient. For other women, magazine articles fulfil the function that might otherwise be fulfilled by a group – they can be reassured that their experiences are 'normal'. As one patient said: 'I'm always reading women's magazines. I love them. I read about the symptoms of the menopause before I had my hysterectomy, so I wasn't too worried. Which was just as well, because at the hospital, no one told me anything.' Another explained: 'If I see any article, I read it to see if I fit in with it, just to console myself.' Another patient, who rarely went to the doctor's, had been persuaded to go by reading a magazine article: 'It helped me, reading those articles where it said you shouldn't soldier on, you should go to your doctor. That was when I was soldiering on.'

Not everyone, however, is 'allowed' access to information on health. One patient described earlier wasn't allowed by her husband to have health literature in the house, because her mother-in-law had had health books and was always 'going on'. And: 'If there's anything on the television about health, my husband makes me turn it off. He says, "that's not entertainment." '

Certainly, some programmes may make viewers anxious. Discussions of illness which start with rather vague general symptoms, or symptoms which in a minor form are common, may send patients to the doctor's next day. But anxieties caused by having a reasonable general knowledge about health and illness are far outweighed by the anxieties of ignorance.

What, then, are the fundaments of change that need to be considered? In many respects, the roles of patient and doctor are predefined, and one is often tempted to think that there are good and bad actors in both roles. But the play itself can't be changed without much wider changes. In so far as change does take place, it needs to take place on both sides. Patients need to be strengthened and GPs educated (in the broadest sense of the word) in a way which enables them to support their patients. This would involve, among other things, a better understanding of what it is to be sick, and what it is to be healthy, as well as a proper understanding that the patient is qualified in ways that the doctor is not. It is she, and not the doctor – however skilled – who knows what it is like to have her particular illness in the context of her particular life. The patient, as well as the doctor, can teach. The doctor, as well as the patient, can learn.

There are, of course, doctors who not only hold such a view

themselves, but who actively promote it. They tend not to be very popular among their colleagues. One of these is Professor Peter Huntingford. In an interview reported in *The Listener*, Huntingford talks about the worst sort of doctor–patient relationship:[18]

> The worst is no doubt where the doctor really believes that he knows what is right for those who seek his help. The next worst is where those seeking help believe that the doctor knows best. . . . I think people ought to challenge the profession and say: 'I want you to treat me as I treat you, namely with respect,' but not with such respect that they cannot say, 'I don't believe what you're saying and I don't like the way that you're doing it. Are there any choices? Why can't I be involved in the choice?' Women and men should be able to do this with their doctor.

As we have seen, however, women do have something – though not very much – to gain by allowing themselves to be defined as ill. It is this that may give them a bit of time off, a chance to stop being the carer and become the cared for. And for some, the chance needs to be snatched. One patient explained:

> 'My husband can't bear it if I'm in bed. If I'm in bed, he thinks I'm going to die on him. He's up and down every two minutes saying, "Aren't you getting up? What's up then?" Not that he's not kind. But the minute I put my feet on the ground, he thinks I must be all right and it's back to work.'

The 'permission' to be ill comes from the doctor. A passage in *The Future General Practitioner* explains: 'Every consultation establishes, maintains, terminates or denies the sick role.'[19] The woman patient *needs* her doctor to confirm that she is ill. Withdrawal is permitted only by sickness. The pity of it is, in most cases, the woman patient is neither treated completely as an adult and equal of the doctor, nor is she allowed the opportunity to regress completely and be cared for like a child. Doctors have the power to define illness and health, and therefore the power to give women time off from *acceptable* trouble by attributing to them *unacceptable* trouble. The circumstances in which doctors will exercise this judgment tells us something about doctors' conceptions of the acceptable limits of domestic dedication. Whether the doctor sees this as temporary relief to sustain the domestic role or intervention to prevent the domestic role becoming intolerable makes little difference to the outcome. Far from being actively oppressive, the doctor is expressing the prevailing 'common-sense' view.

The small benefits to women of the prevailing way of doing things – a little bit of time off – are not much. They are the equivalent of the privilege of having the door opened for you by the man who is being paid twice as much and promoted twice as fast for doing the same job. But nor should they be cast aside without recompense when women take greater control of their own health. They are small alleviations of a domestic and social distribution of power which needs radical change. To that extent, a revolution in women's power over their own health is only part of a wider change. Taking control of our own health involves more than simple changes in the balance of power between women patients and doctors. It also involves a recognition of the fact that there are a lot of ills that the doctor can do nothing about. Indeed, that to go to a doctor if your life is making you miserable defines you as ill rather than angry. If you go to the doctor because you are depressed that your husband is being unfaithful, it is much more likely that the GP will prescribe Librium for you than Bromide for him.

We have seen that the sort of categorisations which doctors in general sustain both obscure the realities of women's lives and create tensions within them. Placed before women are a set a duties and ideals with which their own experience is frequently in painful collision. For the doctor, the difference between the ideal of the household and the reality of domestic life may be no more than a failure of knowledge; for the woman, it becomes an internalised part of the tensions of everyday life. So the women become both the principal sufferers from the demands and contradictions of family life and, at the same time, carry the principal responsibility for nurturing the family – both by being its link with the doctor and by accepting the duty of exploiting that link as little as possible in the interests of being a 'good' patient.

As Ehrenreich and English have argued, we do not simply

want 'more' from medicine (though for many millions of women in the world without the most basic medical care, more is crucial). Rather, 'We want more than "more", we want a new *style*, and we want a new *substance* of medical practice as it relates to women.'[20] 'Medical science', they contend, 'could be a liberating force, giving us real control over our own bodies and power in our lives as health workers.'[21] The question 'whose life is it anyway?' is not one to ask only when we are ready to die. It is just as important to ask it when we want to stay well and happily alive. And there are signs that even the most patient of patients want to see a bit of change.

Appendix

Normally, the appendix, like the notes, tables and graphs, is rather unappetising material in comparison with the main text. I hope that this isn't the case with this one. It consists first of a description of the study from which much of the material in this book is drawn. Second, in order not to break up the text with references and notes, these also appear in the appendix. Finally, there is a brief resource and reading list which relates to each chapter. Much of what appears in this list influenced me in writing the book.

The patients, the practices and the study

The study of women and their doctors on which this book draws took place between 1976 and 1979 and was partially aided by a small grant from the SSRC. The original investigators were Michèle Barrett and myself. The study was designed to examine the high incidence of General Practitioner consultation among women, and particularly among middle-aged women, most of whom are no longer consulting for their children's aches, pains and minor illnesses, few of whom need ante-natal care and large numbers of whom already have their contraceptive needs sorted out. We wanted in particular to look at the significance of the doctor in the lives of his or her female patients.

In order to look at these high consultation rates, and to talk to women and their doctors about their health, we took eight practices in different parts of the country, and from each, selected fifteen 'high' and fifteen 'low' consulters through a tedious process of taking a group of women born between 1921 and 1931 from the age/sex register of the practice, writing to the women, getting permission to look at their records, and then counting the number of consultations. Of those selected, the 'high' consulters were significantly more willing to be interviewed than the 'low' consulters. Not only was it important, of course, to know why some women spent a lot of time at the doctor's, it was also important to know why some women never went, or almost never went; this is why we looked at the low as well as the high consulters. There is a widely held view, which has found currency among the general public as well as the medical profession, that many of the high consulters are going to the doctor's for what are considered to be 'psychosomatic' disorders. Starting from the view that the high consultation rates might well be, at least in part, the product of a woman's social situation, we held that social rather than psychological explanations might well be more useful in looking at this high attendance. Basically, were the problems we were looking at in women's heads, or in their lives?

In order to look at this, and anxious to avoid the bias of looking at only one or two selected practices in our own places of work, the eight practices had a very wide geographical spread, from the south of England to parts of Scotland. In order to maintain confidentiality, the practices cannot be listed here, though some details can be given. Five of the practices were suburban, two inner-city, and one rural. There were two single-handed practices, two partnerships of two and three doctors, and four group practices operating from health centres. The GPs whose practices we used were largely representative of their group – middle-class, middle-aged, white males. However, of the twenty-six doctors working in the eight practices, there were seven women, including a woman trainee, several younger doctors, one elderly doctor and two 'overseas' doctors.

In one respect, the doctors and practices we looked at may have been atypical, and this was in terms of their friendly and helpful tolerance of, and in some cases extreme helpfulness towards, us as sociologists and researchers. Much medical sociology, as the doctors we dealt with were perfectly well aware, challenges fundamental aspects of both the organisation and practice of medicine. Some of our contacts with the practices were made through personal approaches, although none of the doctors themselves were known to us, other than professionally, before we began the study. (Some have become friends subsequently – notwithstanding, in some cases, disagreements about the views which we might hold.)

Of the doctors we approached who declined to take part, most gave as a reason pressure of work, or participation in other projects. One harassed single-handed GP with 3,400 patients on his list wrote that he would be glad to participate and that: 'I feel that we can soon dig up the high consulters, but the low ones may be a little difficult.'

Another GP wrote: 'Sociological stuff interests me, and is really quite well known to most doctors' (it was perhaps for this reason that he withdrew from the study in order to participate in a mammoth Medical Research Council blood pressure trial). He went on to make the important point that 'the conclusions one draws from such [sociological] observations are radically variable depending on your point of view. . . . Speculation is much more fun than specification. . . . However, I'm sure quantification is worth doing.' This particular reservation is worth mentioning since it draws a sharp contrast between 'hard' ('scientific') evidence, and the interpretation of so called 'soft' data. Not only is it easier to interpret the gauge on a sphygmomanometer than it is to interpret what someone says (what someone says is, after all, subjective), the implication is that it is also more valuable. It was not only the GP who was taking part in the blood pressure trial who was worried about the unscientific nature of the sort of research we were doing. One doctor wrote, 'I doubt if I have any useful views. . . . I tend to regard everyone as patients, and not consistently divide them up in categories according to age or sex or anything else.' Another very experienced woman GP wrote: 'my ideas [on women patients] are very personal and not backed up by any scientific data. I rather doubt whether they would be of much use to you'. Given the sort of training which doctors go through, such a view is hardly surprising. Medical education, explicitly at least, is concerned with the clinical and the scientific. But quite apart from the fact that our ideas about what is scientifically 'known' change over time, very large parts of a GP's work, as those who run the training schemes are well aware, is not to do with the scientific tests and clinical observations so carefully learnt during the hospital training, but is an art. So much so, that qualitative evidence of the sort we were seeking is clearly at least as important as knowing what proportions of women visit the doctor's and when.

Our view that the social and emotional component of ill-health should be examined more systematically was by no means new. As early as 1963, D. L. Crombie, the director of the Royal College of General Practitioners' research team in Birmingham was writing of non-organic factors in disease: 'The present (medical) nomenclature produces a distortion notably by underrating the emotional content of disease.' The author had come to this conclusion as the result of a study in which a group of GPs were asked to assess the emotional and organic factors in disease in 100 consecutive patients presenting with 'new' complaints. Instead of assessing emotional factors as relevant to the 5–10 per cent of patients which Crombie had felt to be the usually accepted figure, those participating in the study felt that such factors were far more relevant than had been supposed. When asked to rank the importance of emotional factors in a given illness presented by a patient, the doctors participating felt that its importance equalled the organic in 27 per cent of the cases and was 'appreciable' in a further 21 per cent. The implication drawn was that illness is 'bipartite' in the sense that both organic and emotional factors are involved, and that medical training should encourage students to bear both aspects in mind when making diagnoses. So far so good. But although the Royal College of General Practitioners had found a fair degree of consensus as far as emotional factors were concerned, such was by no means the case when they came to look in a preliminary way at the social component of disease. The doctors participating in the pilot surveys to look at this were far more likely to see social factors as complicating, rather than contributory, forces. Among the individual practitioners participating, views ranged from one doctor who felt that *all* his cases contained social factors, to another who felt that social factors were relevant to none of his patients.

Given this difficulty experienced by doctors in looking at the social factors involved in consultation, one criticism of our research in the medical press was probably misplaced. Commenting on a report of the small grant we had been given to carry out the study, a doctor wrote to the paper: 'I should have thought that any research money would be spent far more effectively on subjects which we *do not* comprehend.'

The influence of social factors on illness and on consultation is clearly very difficult to assess. We did, however, find broad patterns, which have been confirmed elsewhere. But at the end of the day, a good deal of the information we had collected was on areas which had originally been peripheral to our interests (the niceness or otherwise of the doctor, for instance) but clearly central to the interests of the women we were talking to. Researchers frequently complain about the difficulties they have in getting their 'subjects' to respond adequately to certain questions, to understand what is being asked (in the way that the researcher intends questions to be understood), and generally to make the researcher's life easier by giving succinct answers, not straying off the point, and not asking questions back. One of the reasons for this, presumably, is that the world that interests the researcher (or the doctor) is not always the world which interests the person being researched (or patient). The patient/subject of the research, unlike the passive object of scientific research, frequently has ideas of her own concerning what is important. The doctor may wish to discard a lot of such information, since it does not fit in with the 'history' he has been taught to take to diagnose a particular illness. Similarly, the social researcher may be all too tempted to discard the data which do not fit into the elegantly constructed glass slipper of research design. In some cases, these data may not be particularly welcome to the sort of approach being adopted by the researcher, as is abundantly clear from much of the content of this book. Not only do most doctors think they're pretty good chaps, but most of the women patients we spoke to were inclined to share this view. Not only did the doctors have highly stereotyped views of what a woman's role should be, but most of the women we spoke to were only too willing, on one level, to be slotted into such a role.

In short, in many respects, what emerged from the interviews was far richer in areas which mattered to our respondents than it was in areas central to our investigation. Going through the transcripts of interviews, it was striking to see the ways in which the most unpromising of questions could serve as a vehicle for remarks, insights and comments which the women wanted to make about their health and their doctors. Such are the data on which this book has largely relied.

Notes, including resource lists

General reading and general information

This is not a health handbook, so if there are particular health complaints that you would like more information on, it is worth looking at *Our Bodies Ourselves*. This was originally written by a group of American women, but was revised for British readers by Jill Rakusen and Angela Phillips, and is available as a Penguin paperback. As well as giving a lot of useful information, it also gives contact addresses of organisations which can give advice about particular problems.

The Feminist Library and Information Centre (formerly the Women's Research and Resources Centre) is a library which provides information facilities on subjects of importance to women. If you are working on women and health, they have a research index which may help put you in touch with others working in your area. Their address is: Hungerford House, Victoria Embankment, London, WC2 (tel. 01-930 0715). If you are disabled, phone in advance so that help can be arranged with using the ramp. The library is on the first floor, but workers will gladly bring material to A Woman's Place, on the ground floor, for disabled users.

The Women's Health Information Service has recently been set up with the aim of establishing an information service that collects, sifts, clarifies and disseminates health knowledge and information on medical care. Their address is: 52 Featherstone St, London EC1 (tel. 01-251 6580).

Notes and further reading

Chapter 1 Women, the patient patients

A useful introduction to the area of women and medicine, written by two women doctors is: Joyce Leeson and Judith Gray, *Women and Medicine*, Tavistock, 1978.

A collection of articles looking at various issues relevant to the health of women, including contraception, abortion, nurses' training and doctors' training appears in: Helen Roberts (ed.), *Women, Health and Reproduction*, Routledge & Kegan Paul, 1981.

An excellent essay on the impact of feminism on medicine is: Mary Ann Elston, 'Medicine as Old Husbands' Tales', in *Men's Studies Modified*, ed. Dale Spender, Pergamon, 1981.

A recent discussion of women and medicine in Britain which forms part of an Open University course on *The Changing Experience of Women* is: Lesley Doyal and Mary Ann Elston, *Medicine and Health*, Unit 14, Course U221, *The Changing Experience of Women*, Open University, 1983. For more details of the course itself, write to: Open University (Admissions Office), PO Box 48, Walton Hall, Milton Keynes MK7 6AB. For details of how to obtain units, write to: Open University Enterprises, 12 Cotteridge Close, Stony Stratford, Milton Keynes MK11 1BY.

An important sociological account of general practice is Ann Cartwright's *Patients and their Doctors*, Routledge & Kegan Paul, 1967, and, more recently with R. Anderson, *General Practice Revisited*, Tavistock, 1981.

Notes

1 Unless otherwise stated, the quotations which appear in this book come from interviews with doctors and patients and passages taken from case notes as part of the study described in more detail above.
2 See Graham and Oakley (1981).
3 Ehrenreich and English (1974a), p.5.
4 *Wall Street Journal*, vol.CXCV, no.9, 14 January 1980, article by Joanne Lublin.
5 Irving Zola (1972), quoted in Stimson (1975b).
6 H. Lennard *et al.* (1971), pp.18-19, quoted in Stimson (1975b).
7 Karen Dunnell and Ann Cartwright (1971), quoted in Parish (1971).
8 Stimson (1976).

9 For a discussion of statistics on women's health, see Macfarlane (1980), and OPCS (1974) which give details of morbidity statistics from general practice.
10 Nathanson (1975).
11 Gove and Tudor (1973).
12 Janet Finch and Dulcie Groves (1980) set out the arguments and evidence for the view that community care policies rely extensively on women's unpaid labour in the home. A collection of essays they published more recently (Finch and Groves, 1983) discusses women's experience of caring for dependent people.
13 Landau n.d., p.21.
14 Oakley (1980), p.41.
15 Ibid., p.15.
16 Young (1981), p.148.
17 Rakusen (1975), p.7.
18 Madeleine Simms (1979a) gives an historical account of the entry of women to the British medical profession, and (1979b) discusses *A Woman Hater*, a novel by Charles Reade about a young woman's struggle to enter the medical profession in the late nineteenth century.
19 Haspels and Musaph (1979), p.7.

Chapter 2 What do women think of their doctors?

There is not a great deal written on the woman patient's point of view, though a good sociological account of going to see the doctor is provided in: Gerry Stimson and Barbara Webb, *Going to See the Doctor*, Routledge & Kegan Paul, 1975.

Notes

1 Stimson and Webb (1975), p.90.
2 *Woman's Own* 28 January 1961, quoted in White (1970). Barely twenty years later, such an article would be very unlikely to appear.
3 The largest proportion of women GPs are in the category 'trainees and others' as the table below taken from Macfarlane (1980) shows:

Percentage of women among selected grades of full and part time doctors and nurses, England, 1977

Grade	Women (%)
Doctors	
Hospital doctors	18.0
Consultant	9.6
Senior registrar	18.9
Registrar	17.8
Senior house officer	22.9
House officer	30.6
General Practitioners	15.6
Unrestricted principals	14.1
Trainees and others	36.7
Community health	53.8
Community medicine	29.8
Clinical grades	57.9
Hospital nurses and midwives	89.9
Registered nurses	83.3
Student nurses	88.2
Enrolled nurses	90.8
Pupil nurses	92.2
Other nurses	95.1
Midwives	100.0

Source: *Health and Personal Social Services Statistics for England*, 1977.

4 Cartwright and Anderson (1981), quoted in McPherson and Anderson (1983), p.11.
5 McPherson and Anderson (1983), p.11.
6 Young (1981).
7 Quoted from the editorial of the *Lancet*, 3 November 1877, in Simms (1979b).
8 Extract from the *British Medical Journal*, 1877, quoted in *British Medical Journal* (1977).
9 Ibid.

10 Savage and Wilson (1977).
11 Gibson (1981).
12 Ibid., p.69.
13 Consumers' Association (1983), pp.254-7.
14 Oakley (1981), p.276.
15 Ibid., p.280.
16 Oakley, McPherson and Roberts (1984), p.99.
17 Farrell *et al.* (1983b), p.8.
18 Farrell *et al.* (1983a), p.27.
19 Young (1981).

Chapter 3 What do doctors think of their women patients?
It would not be true to say that you can't generalise. The sad fact is that you can. Within the culture of medical schools, of professional bodies within medicine, of medical textbooks, there is a view of 'the patient' which tends not to be very flattering. That said, there are, of course, large numbers of doctors who do treat their patients with the same respect that they get from them. An example of a humane approach, where each patient is related to as an individual can be seen in: John Berger and Jean Mohr (1976), *A Fortunate Man*, Readers & Writers Publishing Co-operative.

Notes
1 Stimson (1976).
2 Ibid., p.56. In fairness, one should point out that some doctors in Stimson's study, did not think of patients in terms of trouble. He writes: 'Answers such as the following, indicating that the doctor did not think of patients in terms of trouble . . . were rare: "I do not look upon patients as giving me trouble. It is my duty and privilege to be troubled and for which I am paid by the state on behalf of my patients" ' (ibid., p.45).
3 Ibid., pp.57–8.
4 Dungal (1978).
5 Friedan (1965).
6 Royal College of General Practitioners (1972).
7 Ibid., p.33.
8 Craddock (1976), p.116.
9 Ibid., pp.123–4.
10 Scully and Bart (1973).

11 Ibid., p.1048, quoting Jeffcoate (1967), p.726.
12 Elston (1981).
13 Jeffcoate (1975), quoted in Elston (1981).
14 Elston (1981), p.v (preface).
15 Ibid., p.190.
16 Jeffcoate (1975), p.568, quoted in Elston (1981).
17 Macdonald (1983).
18 Stimson (1975a), p.265.
19 Private correspondence from faculty member at a British medical school, January 1983. It would be unfair to name the medical school that has the courage to carry out such an investigation!
20 For a brief, sympathetic and clear description of the Balint approach, see Cunningham (1975). For Balint's own description of his approach, see Balint (1970). Significantly, perhaps, the title is *The Doctor, His* [sic] *Patient and the Illness.*
21 Stimson and Webb (1975), pp.142-3, quoting Balint *et al.* (1970), p.xiv.
22 Tunnadine (1970), pp.2-3.

Chapter 4 What makes you ill? Old wives' tales versus old doctors' tales

An excellent and very readable book on the experts' advice to women is: Barbara Ehrenreich and Deirdre English (1979), *For Her Own Good*, Pluto Press. It reassesses 150 years of advice (from social scientists as well as doctors!) and shows how the experts have usurped women's own skills – justifying their efforts by saying that it is 'for her own good'.

See also: Barbara Ehrenreich and Deirdre English (1974a), *Complaints and Disorders: The Sexual Politics of Sickness*, and Barbara Ehrenreich and Deirdre English (1974b), *Witches, Midwives and Nurses: A History of Women Healers*. Both are published by Compendium, which has a bookshop at 240 Camden High Street, London NW1.

Notes

1 Graham and Oakley (1981).
2 Titmuss (1968), quoted in Cartwright and O'Brien (1975), maintained, 'We have learnt from fifteen years' experience of the Health Service that the higher income groups know how to make better use of the Service; they tend to receive more specialist attention; occupy

more of the beds in better equipped and staffed hospitals; receive more elective surgery; have better maternity care; are more likely to get psychiatric help and psychotherapy than low income groups – particularly the unskilled.' Although Cartwright and O'Brien were not convinced by the evidence Titmuss had used in support of his argument, they themselves conclude: 'There appears to us to be fairly conclusive evidence that the middle class make more use of preventative services. There is also enough evidence to suggest that the middle class may, in relation to a number of services, receive better care' (p.93).

3 See *The General Household Survey* (1974). The table on self-reported morbidity and GP consultations by sex, age and marital status indicates that unmarried women consult less than either married or formerly married women.
4 Ivan Reid (1982), p.38.
5 Strong (1979).
6 Armitage *et al.* (1979).
7 Achte (1970), p.8.
8 Ibid., p.8.
9 Landau n.d.
10 Ibid., foreword.
11 Ibid., p.30.
12 Parish (1971), p.10.
13 Ibid.
14 Ibid., p.22.
15 Ibid., p.33.
16 Stimson (1975b), p.156.
17 Ibid., p.157.
18 Ibid., p.157.
19 Stimson (1975a), p.267.
20 Landau n.d., p.21.
21 Achte (1970), p.8.
22 Ibid., p.18.

Chapter 5 Family matters

Three of Ann Oakley's books: *Housewife* (Allen Lane, 1974), *Becoming a Mother* (Martin Robertson, 1979) and *Subject Women* (Penguin, 1982) give many insights into the relationships between family life and work, and the health of women. The final chapter of her book *Women*

Confined (Martin Robertson, 1980) takes the brave step of making concrete proposals concerning birth, bringing up children and the wider context which might enable women to have an increased sense of achievement and self-determination.

Notes

1 This quotation comes from Susan Griffin's beautiful poetry play, *Voices* (Griffin, 1975). I am grateful to Susan Griffin for her permission to use it, and to Pauline Bart for drawing it to my attention.
2 Elliott Binns (1973), p.256.
3 Royal College of General Practitioners (1972), p.157.
4 Stimson and Webb (1975), p.98.
5 Royal College of General Practitioners (1972), p.15.
6 For a discussion concerning the length of time spent in marriage by men and women, see Burkitt and Rose (1981).

Chapter 6 Making changes

For a discussion of the broader political changes that need to be made in our health system, see: Lesley Doyal (with Imogen Pennell), *The Political Economy of Health*, Pluto, 1979.

For more information on those involved in practical moves to make changes, contact the Women's Health Information Centre.

Notes

1 Oakley (1982), p.81.
2 Speech given at a conference organised by the World Health Organization and the Scottish Health Education Group, May 1983.
3 Wimpole (1976).
4 Pickering (1978), p.33.
5 See Chapter 2, note 3.
6 Editorial, *British Medical Journal*, 10 January 1976, p.56.
7 Sprackling (1976).
8 *British Medical Journal*, 10 January 1976, p.56.
9 Bewley and Bewley (1975), p.270.
10 Advertisement from *The Times Health Supplement*, 6 November 1981.
11 This does not mean that some do not attempt to do so, simply that it is rarely a part of their work or an item for which they are paid. It

is significant that much of such education as there is appears largely designed to lessen demands on the doctor rather than to increase the autonomy of the patient.

12 Electroconvulsive therapy (ECT) involves passing an electric current through the brain, by means of electrodes attached to a patient's temple. Used mainly for seriously depressed patients, it is held that ECT can remove the symptoms of depression in some patients.

13 Carsten Jespersen, personal communication.

14 See Oakley, McPherson and Roberts (1984).

15 These are taken from an unpublished paper by Dr Katy Gardner, a Liverpool GP. See also Gardner (1981), 'Well Woman Clinics: a Positive Approach to Women's Health'.

16 Gardner, unpublished paper p.3.

17 Phillips and Rakusen (1978).

18 Huntingford (1975), p.815.

19 Royal College of General Practitioners (1972), p.9.

20 Ehrenreich and English (1974b), p.84.

21 Ehrenreich and English (1974a), p.40.

Bibliography

Achte, K. (1970), 'Menopause from the psychiatrist's point of view', in *Acta Obstetrica et Gynaecologica Scandinavia*, vol.49, suppl.1.

Armitage, K.J. *et al.* (1979), 'Response of Physicians to Medical Complaints in Men and Women', *Journal of the American Medical Association*, 18 May, pp.2186-7.

Balint, M., (1970), *The Doctor, His Patient, and the Illness*, London, Pitman Medical.

Balint, J., Hunt, J., Joyce, D., Marinker, M., and Woodcock, J. (1970). *Treatment or Diagnosis: A Study of Repeat Prescriptions in General Practice*, London, Tavistock.

Barrett, M. and Roberts, H. (1978), 'Doctors and their Patients: The Social Control of Women in General Practice' in C. and B. Smart (eds), *Women, Sexuality and Social Control*, London, Routledge & Kegan Paul.

Berger, John and Mohr, Jean (1976), *A Fortunate Man*, London, Readers & Writers Publishing Co-operative.

Bewley, Beulah R. and Bewley, Thomas H. (1975), 'Hospital Doctors' Career Structure and Misuse of Medical Womanpower' *Lancet*, 9 August, pp.270-2.

Bowlby, John (1953), *Child Care and the Growth of Love*, Harmondsworth, Penguin.

British Medical Journal (1977), Extract from the *British Medical Journal* 1877 (n.d.), p.1149, 30 April.

Burkitt, B. and Rose, H. (1981), 'Why be a Wife?' *Sociological Review*, vol.29, no.1, February, pp.67-76.

Cartwright, A. (1967), *Patients and their Doctors*, London, Routledge & Kegan Paul.

Cartwright, A. and Anderson, R. (1981), *General Practice Revisited*, London Tavistock.

Cartwright, A. and O'Brien, M. (1975), 'Social Class Variations in Health Care and in the Nature of General Practitioner Consultations', in M. Stacey (ed.), *The Sociology of the National Health Service*, Sociological Review Monograph No. 22, University of Keele, pp.77-98.

Consumers' Association (1983), *A Patient's Guide to the NHS*, London, Consumers' Association and Hodder & Stoughton.

Craddock, Dennis (1976), *A Short Textbook of General Practice*, London, H.K. Lewis and Co. Ltd.

Crombie, D.L. (1963), 'The Procrustean Bed of Medical Nomenclature, *Lancet*, 1 June, pp.1205-6.

Cunningham, John (1975), 'Powerful Doses of the Doctor', *New Psychiatry*, 16 January, pp.14-15.

Doyal, Lesley (with Imogen Pennell) (1979), *The Political Economy of Health*, London, Pluto.

Doyal, Lesley and Elston, Mary Ann (1983), *Medicine and Health*, Unit 14, Course U221, *The Changing Experience of Women*, Milton Keynes, Open University Enterprises.

Dungal, Leifur (1978), 'Physicians' Responses to Patients: A Study of Factors Involved in the Office Interview', *Journal of Family Practice*, vol.6, no.5, pp.1065-73.

Dunnell, Karen and Cartwright, Ann (1971), *Medicine Takers, Prescribers and Hoarders*, London, Routledge & Kegan Paul.

Ehrenreich, Barbara and English, Deirdre (1974a), *Complaints and Disorders: The Sexual Politics of Sickness*, London, Compendium.

Ehrenreich, Barbara and English, Deirdre (1974b), *Witches, Midwives and Nurses: A History of Women Healers*, London, Compendium.

Ehrenreich, Barbara and English, Deirdre (1979), *For Her Own Good*, London, Pluto.

Elliott Binns, C.P. (1973), 'An Analysis of Lay Medicine', *Journal of the Royal College of General Practitioners*, vol.23, pp.255-640.

Elston, Mary Ann (1981), 'Medicine as Old Husbands' Tales', in Dale Spender (ed.), *Men's Studies Modified*, London, Pergamon.

Farrell, C., Humphrey, C., Smith, C.W.L., and Hindley, C.P. (1983a), *Evaluation of Maternity Care in General Practice: Second Report*, Department of Applied Social Studies, Polytechnic of North London.

Farrell, C. *et al.* (1983b), *Evaluation of Maternity Care in General Practice: Final Report*, Department of Applied Social Studies, Polytechnic of North London.

Finch, Janet and Groves, Dulcie (1980), 'Community Care and the Family: A Case for Equal Opportunities?' *Journal of Social Policy*, vol.9, no.4, pp.487-511.

Finch, Janet and Groves, Dulcie (eds) (1983), *Women, Work and Caring*, London, Routledge & Kegan Paul.

Friedan, Betty (1965), *The Feminine Mystique*, Harmondsworth, Penguin.

Gardner, Katy (1981), 'Well Women Clinics: A Positive Approach to Women's Health', in Helen Roberts (ed.), *Women, Health and Reproduction*, London, Routledge & Kegan Paul.

General Household Survey (1974), OPCS Social Survey Division, London, HMSO.

Gibson, Roland (1981), *The Family Doctor, His Life and History*, London, Allen & Unwin.

Gove, W.R. and Tudor, J. (1973), 'Adult Sex Roles and Mental Illness', *American Journal of Sociology*, vol.78, p.812.

Graham, Hilary and Oakley, Ann (1981), 'Competing Ideologies of Reproduction: Medical and Maternal Perspectives in Pregnancy', in Helen Roberts (ed.) *Women, Health and Reproduction*, London, Routledge & Kegan Paul.

Griffin, Susan (1975), *Voices*, New York, The Feminist Press.

Haspels, A.A. and Musaph, H. (eds), *Psychosomatics in Perimenopause*, Lancaster, MTP Press.

HMSO (1983), *Patients' Rights: A Guide for NHS Patients and Doctors*, London, HMSO.

Huntingford, P. (1975), 'Does the Doctor Know Best – a Professional

Opinion,' *The Listener*, 18 December, p.815.

Jeffcoate, Norman (1967), *Principles of Gynaecology*, London, Butterworth.

Jeffcoate, Norman (1975), *Principles of Gynaecology* (4th edn), London, Butterworth.

Landau, M.E. (n.d.), *So Now You Know About the Change of Life*, London, The British Medical Association.

Leeson, Joyce and Gray, Judith (1978), *Women and Medicine*, London, Tavistock.

Lennard, H. *et al.* (1971), *Mystification and Drug Misuse*, San Francisco, Jossey Bass.

Macdonald, Rosemary (1983), 'Personal View', *British Medical Journal*, 19 November p.1544.

Macfarlane, Alison (1980), 'Official Statistics on Women's Health and Illness', *EOC Research Bulletin*, no.4, autumn, pp.43-77, Manchester, Equal Opportunities Commission.

McPherson, Ann and Anderson, Anne (eds) (1983), *Women's Problems in General Practice*, Oxford University Press.

Nathanson, C. (1975), 'Illness and the Feminine Role: A Theoretical Review', *Social Science and Medicine*, vol.9, pp.57-62.

Oakley, Ann (1974), *Housewife*, London, Allen Lane.

Oakley, Ann (1979), *Becoming a Mother*, Oxford, Martin Robertson.

Oakley, Ann (1980), *Women Confined*, Oxford, Martin Robertson.

Oakley, Ann (1981), *From Here to Maternity*, Harmondsworth, Penguin.

Oakley, Ann (1982), *Subject Women*, Harmondsworth, Penguin.

Oakley, Ann, McPherson, Ann and Roberts, Helen (1984), *Miscarriage*, London, Fontana.

OPCS (1974), *Morbidity Statistics from General Practice, Second National Morbidity Study 1970-71*, London, HMSO.

Parish, Peter A. (1971), 'The Prescribing of Psychotropic Drugs in General Practice', *Journal of the Royal College of General Practitioners*, supplement no. 4, vol.21, no.92.

Pereira, Gray D.J. (1982), *Training for General Practice*, London, Macdonald & Evans.

Phillips, Angela and Rakusen, Jill (eds of British edn) (1978), *Our Bodies Ourselves*, Harmondsworth, Penguin.

Pickering, George (1978), *Quest for Excellence in Medical Education*, Oxford University Press.

Rakusen, Jill (1975), 'The Pill Report: Information or Propaganda?' *Spare Rib*, no.32, pp.6-8.

Reid, Ivan (1982), 'Vital statistics' in Reid, Ivan and Wormald, Eileen, *Sex Differences in Britain*, Grant McIntyre, London.

Roberts, Helen (ed.) (1981), *Women, Health and Reproduction*, London, Routledge & Kegan Paul.

Royal College of General Practitioners (1972), *The Future General Practitioner, Learning and Teaching*, London, Royal College of General Practitioners.

Savage, Richard and Wilson, Ann (1977), 'Doctors' Attitudes to Women in Medicine', *Journal of the Royal College of General Practitioners*, vol.27, pp.363-5.

Scully, Diana and Bart, Pauline (1973), 'A Funny Thing Happened to Me on the Way to the Orifice: Women in Gynaecology Textbooks', *American Journal of Sociology*, vol.78, no.4, pp.1045-9.

Simms, Madeleine (1979a), 'The Medical Woman Question', *World Medicine*, February 24.

Simms, Madeleine (1979b), 'A Woman Hater', *Spare Rib*, no.85, August, pp.18-20.

Sprackling, M.E. (1976), letter to the *British Medical Journal*, 7 February, p.339.

Stimson, Gerry V. (1975a), 'Women in a Doctored World', *New Society*, 1 May, pp.265-7.

Stimson, Gerry V. (1975b), 'The Message of Psychotropic Drug Ads', *Journal of Communication*, vol.25, no.3, pp.153-60.

Stimson, Gerry V. (1976), 'General Practitioners: Trouble and Types of Patients', in Margaret Stacey (ed.), *The Sociology of the NHS*, Sociological Review Monograph No. 22, University of Keele.

Stimson, Gerry V. and Webb, Barbara (1975), *Going to See the Doctor*, London, Routledge & Kegan Paul.

Strong, P. (1979), *The Ceremonial Order of the Clinic*, London, Routledge & Kegan Paul.

Titmuss, Richard M. (1968), *Commitment to Welfare*, London, Allen & Unwin.

Tunnadine, L.P.D. (1970), *Contraception and Sexual Life*, London, Tavistock.

White, Cynthia (1970), *Women's Magazines 1693-1968*, London, Michael Joseph.

Wimpole, Roderick (1976), 'Doctor's Diary',*Woman's Own*, 28 August.

Young, Gail (1981), 'A Woman in Medicine: Reflections from the Inside', in Helen Roberts (ed.), *Women, Health and Reproduction*, London, Routledge & Kegan Paul.

Zola, Irving (1972), 'Medicine as an Institution of Social Control', *Sociological Review*, vol.20, no.4, pp.487-504.

Index

P A N D O R A P R E S S

an imprint of Routledge and Kegan Paul

For further information about Pandora Press books, please write to the Mailing List Dept at Pandora Press, 14 Leicester Square, London WC2H 7PH or in the USA at 9 Park Street, Boston, Mass. 02108; or in Australia at 464 St Kilda Road, Melbourne, Victoria 3004, Australia.

Some Pandora titles you may enjoy:

WOMEN'S HISTORY IN SHORT STORIES

DARING TO DREAM

Utopian stories by United States women: 1836-1919

Compiled, edited and introduced by Carol Farley Kessler

Carol Farley Kessler has unearthed an extraordinary assortment of visionary writing, writings which encapsulate all the yearnings of a vanished generation for a future which has still to be made. Some women write with irony, describing journeys through time and space to parallel but inverted worlds where sober-suited women run commerce and affairs of state while men either prink and preen in beribboned breeches, or are weakened by the burden of unending housework. Other writers lay out complicated blueprints for a non-sexist society. One woman dreams, touchingly, of a fantastic future where men get up in the night to comfort crying children. The stories demonstrate that even in the early nineteenth century women were arguing that male and female 'character traits' were the product of their roles, not of their biology; and they make apparent the hidden roots of the discontent, longing and anger which was later to erupt in the great movements of women for change.

MY COUNTRY IS THE WHOLE WORLD

an anthology of women's work on peace and war

Cambridge Women's Peace Collective (eds)

Women's struggle for peace is no recent phenomenon. In this book, the work of women for peace from 600 BC to the present is documented in a unique collection of extracts from songs, poems, diaries, letters, petitions, pictures, photographs and pamphlets through the ages. A book to give as a gift, to read aloud from, to research from, to teach from, *My Country is the Whole World* is both a resource and an inspiration for all who work for peace today.

'An historic document . . . readers will be amazed at the extent of the collection.' *Labour Herald*

'A beautifully presented and illustrated book which makes for accessible and enlightening reading.' *Morning Star*

0-86358-004-1 Social Questions/History 306pp A5 illustrated throughout paperback

DISCOVERING WOMEN'S HISTORY

a practical manual

Deirdre Beddoe

Rainy Sunday afternoons, long winter evenings: why not set yourself a research project, either on your own or in a group or classroom? This is the message from Deirdre Beddoe, an historian who tears away the mystique of her own profession in this step-by-step guide to researching the lives of ordinary women in Britain from 1800 to 1945. *Discovering Women's History* tells you how to get started on the detective trail of history and how to stalk your quarry through attics and art galleries, museums and old newspapers, church archives and the Public Records Office – and how to publish your findings once you have completed your project.

'An invaluable and fascinating guide to the raw material for anyone approaching this unexplored territory.' *The Sunday Times*

'Thrilling and rewarding and jolly good fun.' *South Wales Argus*

0-86358-008-4 Hobbies/Social History 232pp 198 × 129 mm illustrated